Key advances in the effective management

of

Myocardial Infarction

Edited by

D Holdright and A Timmis

Series Organizer

A Miles

Proceedings of a symposium sponsored by Merck, Sharp & Dohme Ltd and held at the Royal Society of Medicine, London, 16th September 1998

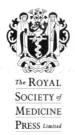

The ROYAL
SOCIETY *of*
MEDICINE
PRESS *Limited*

1 Wimpole Street, London W1M 8AE, UK
207 E. Westminster Road, Lake Forest, IL 60045, USA
http://www.roysocmed.ac.uk

These proceedings are published by the Royal Society of Medicine Press Ltd with financial support from the sponsor. The contributors are responsible for the scientific content and for the views expressed, which are not necessarily those of the editor of the series or of the volume, of the Royal Society of Medicine or of the Royal Society of Medicine Press Ltd. Distribution has been in accordance with the wishes of the sponsor but a copy is available to any fellow of the society at a privileged price.

British Library Cataloguing in Publication Data

A catalogue record for this book is available from the British Library

ISBN 1–85315–390–7

Typeset by Saxon Graphics Ltd, Derby

Printed in Great Britain by Redwood Books, Trowbridge, Wiltshire

Editors

Dr Diana Holdright
The Middlesex Hospital, UCL Hospitals, Mortimer Street, London W1N 8AA

Dr Adam Timmis
London Chest Hospital, Bonner Road, London E2 9JX

Contributors

Dr John Ferguson
Prescription Pricing Authority, Bridge House, 152 Pilgrim Street,
Newcastle-upon-Tyne NE1 6SN

Dr Jane Flint
Dudley Group of Hospitals NHS Trust, West Midlands DY8 5QX

Professor Keith Fox
Cardiovascular Research Unit, Cardiology,
The Royal Infirmary of Edinburgh, Edinburgh EH3 9YW

Dr Manish Gandhi
Wessex Cardiothoracic Centre, Southampton University Hospitals,
Tremona Road, Southampton SO16 6YD

Dr Anthony Gershlick
Department of Academic Cardiology, Glenfield General Hospital,
Leicester LE3 9QP

Dr Caroline Morrison
Greater Glasgow Health Board, Dalian House, PO Box 15329,
350 St Vincent Street, Glasgow G3 8YZ

Dr Michael Schachter
Department of Clinical Pharmacology, Imperial College School of Medicine,
St Mary's Hospital, Norfolk Place, London W2 1PG

Professor Richard Vincent
Cardiac Department, Royal Sussex County Hospital, Eastern Road,
Brighton BN2 5BE

Contents

Foreword

The Key Advances symposia held at the Royal Society of Medicine aim to provide a solidly clinical contribution to evidence-based medicine in the UK. Attention is focused on open debate and the contextual interpretation of new medical evidence in a variety of common disease states.

The symposia are intended to facilitate true analysis of the available evidence: practice guidelines, scientific evidence, cost-effectiveness and clinical audit data.

This book presents clinical strategies for the efficient and effective management of myocardial infarction. The Guest Editors and contributors, all distinguished clinicians in their field, are to be commended for their efforts in producing an accessible, highly readable text of immediate relevance to continuing medical education and personal clinical practice.

Professor Andrew Miles
Series Organizer
St Bartholomew's Hospital, London

Preface

There have been many advances in the management of myocardial infarction in recent years, prompting publication of a Key Advances series addressing this area. Ischaemic heart disease is the single greatest killer in developed countries and is of increasing importance in developing countries, such that any small advance in management generally translates into significant health benefit.

The publication has been designed to cover all the important areas of management in myocardial infarction. The initial chapters address the scale of the problem and aspects of pre-hospital care, which is so frequently overlooked and yet is the period when most fatalities following acute myocardial infarction occur. Subsequent chapters deal with the hospital phase of management, providing a succinct and up-to-date account of modern practice. There follows an informative account detailing the investigation of patients, both in the hospital phase and in the community. The final chapters are devoted to the various aspects of secondary prevention, covering rehabilitation, drug therapy, the role of general practice and the economics of best practice.

This book is a highly readable account of the management of acute myocardial infarction, which will be of particular interest to all practitioners looking after patients with ischaemic heart disease.

Dr Diana Holdright
Consultant Cardiologist
The Middlesex Hospital
London

Scale of the problem

Adam Timmis, London Chest Hospital, London

Coronary heart disease (CHD) is the most common cause of premature death for men and women both in the UK and worldwide, and a substantial proportion of these coronary deaths are the direct result of acute myocardial infarction (MI).[1] Figure 1 shows deaths from all causes and at all ages during 1987 in England and Wales and deaths from CHD broken down according to age.[2] The data show that CHD accounted for nearly one-third of all male deaths and one-quarter of all female deaths. Importantly, a large proportion of these deaths occurred in men and women under the age of 75.

Disease prevalence

The data are similar across a broad range of developed countries, including the US, Australia, Germany and Canada. Encouragingly, however, all these countries have seen a downward trend in coronary mortality in recent years, possibly attributable to increasing public awareness of the importance of lifestyle (particularly smoking, diet and exercise) in the pathogenesis of disease. This downward trend has not been universal however and, in some Eastern European countries, mortality rates from CHD have continued to increase.[3] Reliable data for less developed countries are not available but there is general agreement that, in most, the prevalence of CHD is rising steeply, threatening to overtake malnutrition and infectious disease as the major cause of mortality. The global view, therefore, provides little room for complacency and the decline in coronary mortality occurring in the Western world is almost certainly being balanced by corresponding increments in the Eastern European countries and the developing world.

Although the UK decline in coronary mortality is encouraging, it has not been a uniform pattern. In people of South Asian origin, for example, coronary mortality is continuing to rise (Table 1) posing an important challenge to all concerned in the treatment of MI.[4] The susceptibility of South Asians to coronary artery disease has been difficult to explain in terms of conventional risk factors. There is growing consensus that it is the result of the genetically-determined insulin resistance syndrome; this is characterized by central obesity, hyperinsulinaemia, hypertriglyceridaemia, reduced plasma high density lipoprotein cholesterol and hypertension with or without non-insulin dependent diabetes.[5] Not only are South Asians more susceptible to CHD and MI but case fatality rates are also higher, due largely to the increased prevalence of diabetes in this group.[6] The problem of CHD in the UK South Asian population shows no sign of abating; it is unlikely to be resolved until our understanding of the pathogenic mechanisms improves, so that specific treatment can be applied to reduce the risk.

Figure 1: Deaths from all causes during 1987 in England and Wales and deaths from CHD according to age[2]

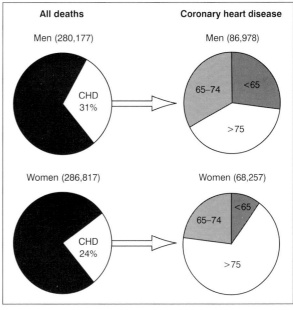

All deaths — Men (280,177) — CHD 31%

Coronary heart disease — Men (86,978) — 65–74, <65, >75

All deaths — Women (286,817) — CHD 24%

Coronary heart disease — Women (68,257) — 65–74, <65, >75

Causes and treatment

There is now general agreement that acute MI is caused by rupture of a coronary atheromatous plaque which provides a stimulus for platelet aggregation and occlusive thrombosis.[7] Acute MI is fatal in about 50% of cases and about one-half of these deaths occur outside hospital very early after coronary occlusion.[8] The majority of these out-of-hospital deaths are attributable to ventricular fibrillation, emphasizing the importance of early access to a defibrillator. In patients admitted to hospital, arrhythmic death is unusual and the major determinant of outcome is infarct size — those with large infarcts and pump failure being at greatest risk.[9]

The benefits of thrombolytic therapy and aspirin in reducing hospital mortality from acute MI are largely attributable to restoration of coronary patency and reduction in infarct size. Five major randomized trials have confirmed that thrombolytic therapy reduces early mortality in patients with acute MI, raising the expectation that application of this treatment would lead to substantial reductions in overall coronary mortality.[10–4] Certainly, a local analysis of coronary care unit (CCU) mortality rates in an East London CCU, before and after introduction of thrombolytic therapy, provided grounds for optimism. Hospital mortality rates fell from 24% to 12%, with concurrent reductions in cardiogenic shock and diuretic requirements, implying that morbidity as well as mortality could be favourably influenced by this type of treatment.[15]

It is important to recognize, however, that hospital mortality rates comprise only a small percentage of overall infarct mortality in acute MI. In addition, while there is general agreement that patients who receive thrombolytic and aspirin therapy derive benefit from it, it is important to consider that those who are ineligible for treatment — about 50% of the infarct population treated in hospital,[16] plus the large numbers who die out of hospital — will derive no benefit.

These considerations almost certainly account for the increasing realization that hospital mortality rates from acute MI have shown appreciable decline only in centres where treatment rates can be maintained at a high level. In the majority of centres with treatment rates of ≤50%, little impact on overall hospital mortality can be expected. Consequently, the population mortality from MI has scarcely been affected by treatment which fails to impact upon the substantial risk from primary ventricular fibrillation, for which early access to a defibrillator is the only remedy of any value.

Conclusion

In the future, the ongoing development of more effective preventive strategies is widely recognized as the the key to achieving further reductions in mortality from CHD and acute MI. This, in turn, will depend upon continuing research, to increase our understanding of the pathogenic mechanisms of the atherosclerotic process. Secondary prevention is, of course, the responsibility of the physician, who should give formal lifestyle advice to every coronary patient and prescribe, as appropriate, those drugs (aspirin, β-blockers, angiotensin-converting enzyme inhibitors and statins) that are known to reduce the risk of recurrent coronary events.

Primary prevention is more difficult and, although the physician may contribute by targeting high-risk subgroups, a population approach requires the intervention of governmental, rather

Table 1 Mortality from coronary heart disease in England and Wales by country of birth: 1970–2 vs 1979–83[3]

Country of birth	% change in standardized mortality ratio		Country of birth	% change in standardized mortality ratio	
	Men	Women		Men	Women
Scotland	−10	−4	Old Commonwealth	−17	−23
Ireland	1	−2	West Europe	−8	−7
Caribbean Commonwealth	−8	−15	US	−23	−36
African Commonwealth	−3	ND	Indian subcontinent	6	13

ND – no data

than medical, agencies. Unfortunately, the available evidence indicates that physicians are not performing well in their delivery of secondary prevention. Even worse are the government agencies who, by failing to ban cigarette advertising while presiding over a massive increase in cigarette consumption in the developing world, are clearly failing to mount an adequate challenge to the ravages of CHD.

References

1. Tunstall-Pedoe H, Kuulasmaa K, Amouyel P *et al*. Myocardial infarctions and coronary deaths in the World Health Organization MONICA Project. Registration Procedures, event rates and case fatality rates in 38 populations from 21 countries in four continents. *Circulation* 1994; **90**: 583–612.

2. Data from the Office of Population Censuses and Surveys Monitor, 1988

3. Sans S, Kesteloot H, Kromhout D, The burden of cardiovascular diseases mortality in Europe. Task force of the European Society of Cardiology on cardiovascular mortality and morbidity statistics in Europe. *Eur Heart J* 1997; **18**: 1231–48.

4. Balarajan R. Ethnic differences in mortality from ischaemic heart disease and cerebrovascular disease in England and Wales. *BMJ* 1991; **302**: 560–4.

5. McKeigue PM, Shah B, Marmot MG. Relation of central obesity and insulin resistance with high diabetes prevalence and cardiovascular risk in South Asians. *Lancet* 1991; **337**: 382–6.

6. Wilkinson P, Sayer J, Laji K *et al*. Comparison of case fatality in South Asian and white patients following acute myocardial infarction. *BMJ* 1996; **312**: 1330–3.

7. Davies MJ, Thomas AC. Plaque fissuring: the cause of acute myocardial infarction, sudden ischaemic death, and crescendo angina. *Br Heart J* 1983; **50**: 127–34.

8. Gandhi M. Clinical epidemiology of coronary heart disease in the UK. *Br J Hosp Med* 1997; **58**: 23–7.

9. Stevenson R, Ranjadayalan K, Wilkinson P *et al*. Short- and long-term prognosis of acute myocardial infarction since introduction of thrombolysis. *BMJ* 1993; **307**: 349–53.

10. Gruppo Italiano per lo Studio della Streptochinasi nell'Infarcto miocardico (GISSI). Effectiveness of intravenous thrombolytic treatment in acute myocardial infarction. *Lancet* 1986; **1**: 397–402.

11. ISAM study group. A prospective trial of intravenous streptokinase in acute myocardial infarction (ISAM). Mortality, morbidity, and infarct size at 21 days. *N Engl J Med* 1986; **314**: 1465–71.

12. ISIS-2 collaborative group. Randomized trial of intravenous streptokinase, oral aspirin, both, or neither, among 17,187 cases of suspected acute myocardial infarction: ISIS-2. *Lancet* 1988; **2**: 349–60.

13. Wilcox RG, Von der Lippe G, Olsen CG *et al*, for the ASSET Study Group. Trial of tissue plasminogen activator for mortality reduction in acute myocardial infarction. Anglo-Scandinavian Study of Early Thrombolysis (ASSET). *Lancet* 1988; **2**: 525–30.

14. AIMS Trial Study Group. Effect of intravenous APSAC on mortality after acute myocardial infarction: preliminary report of a placebo-controlled clinical trial. *Lancet* 1988; **1**: 545–9.

15. Ranjadayalan K, Umachandran V, Timmis AD. The clinical impact of introducing thrombolytic and aspirin therapy into the management policy of a coronary care unit. *Am J Med* 1992; **92**: 233–8.

16. French JK, Williams BF, Hart HH *et al*. Prospective evaluation of eligibility for thrombolytic therapy in acute myocardial infarction. *BMJ* 1996; **312**:1637–41.

Pre-hospital care

Richard Vincent, Royal Sussex County Hospital, Brighton

Myocardial infarction (MI) strikes in the community — at home, at work, or while out — usually observed, but often remote from immediate medical care. Management of an attack is initially determined by the actions of the patient or bystander and, subsequently, by the professionals summoned to help. A convenient time-line of care is shown in Figure 1. Indicative times are shown for patient delay, professional delay, time on site with the patient before transportation, transportation delay and the 'door-to-needle' time for administering thrombolysis after arrival at hospital.

Driven by imperatives from studies of the natural history, pathophysiology and treatment of acute MI, a topic that continues to be of practical concern is reducing the delay in receiving professional care. Of equal concern is exploring how such care can, in practice, include all that has been shown to preserve life, limit myocardial damage and ensure comfort during the most crucial phase of the attack.

Imperatives for reducing delay

Epidemiology and natural history

Studies in Europe and the US over the past 35 years give an unvarying account, not only of the high total mortality from ischaemic heart disease, but also of the formidable attrition rate from MI within the first few hours of symptom onset.[1–6] On average, one-third of all cases of MI are fatal before admission to hospital and most of these deaths occur within the first hour.[4,5]

Recent data from Augsberg (one of the participating centres in the MONICA study[4]) provide a clear illustration of the problem (Figure 2a).[7] The overall 28-day fatality rate in 3,729 cases of acute MI in patients aged 24–74 was 58%. Death claimed 28% of all cases within the first hour and 40% within the first four hours.

Of all deaths caused by MI, 60% occur outside hospital and, of these, only 10% are seen by a doctor; 60% are not even witnessed. Data from the UK Heart Attack Study, of 1,234 patients in three British centres,[6] reveals a similar picture. Overall, 75% of the fatalities recorded died before hospital admission but, as illustrated in Figure 2b, within this proportion there was prominent variation with age. For patients <50 years, pre-hospital deaths accounted for 90% of fatalities, but this figure fell to 50% for those aged 70–74.

Pathophysiology

Abrupt instability of an atheromatous coronary plaque is now well-recognized to be the precipitating event in most cases of acute MI.[8] Progressive clot formation at the site of plaque rupture, intra-plaque haemorrhage, accentuated coronary spasm and adventitial inflammation all contribute to coronary occlusion. Embolization to distal coronary vessels may

*Figure 1:
A time-line
(minutes)
representing the
key stages of pre-
hospital care in
acute MI.*

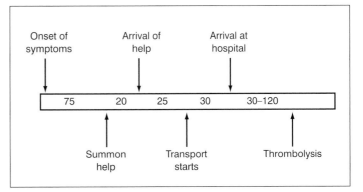

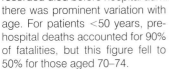

The numbers give an indicative median delay for each stage. Note, however, that there is wide variation in individual patient delay and between the median delays recorded in different studies[20,21,28]

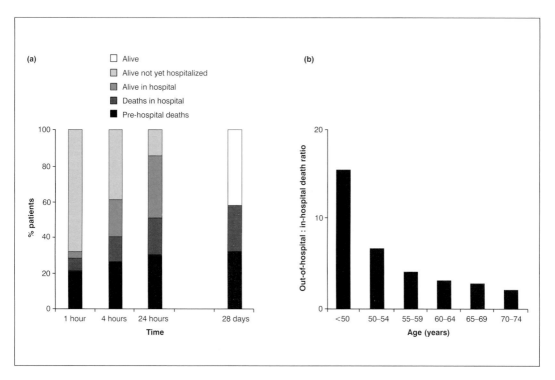

Figure 2:
The high attrition
rate from acute MI
before hospital
admission a)
Fatality pattern in
3,729 cases of
acute MI[7] b) The
effect of age on
the place of death
following an acute
coronary event
expressed as out-
of-hospital: in-
hospital deaths[6]

further jeopardize myocardial perfusion; in addition the process of acute coronary obstruction is dynamic and fluctuating. Initial progression is common, not only by clot propagation, but by progressive cross-linking between fibrin strands; in addition, as a clot stabilizes, it becomes increasingly resistant to the action of thrombolytic agents.

In the myocardium supplied by the occluding artery, a rapid and progressive change takes place, initially of function and then of structure.[9] In experimental animals, necrosis advances in a 'wavefront' pattern for about six hours following coronary occlusion,[10] a pattern also likely to apply to man. The important therapeutic implication of this observation — as confirmed in the experimental model — is that there is a short, finite time-window during which myocardium may be salvaged by reperfusion (Figure 3a).[10] Other early events in the evolution of acute MI include the local release of potassium and catecholamines and marked auto-nomic instability.[11] This potent combination readily predisposes to the ventricular arrhythmias that remain responsible for the majority of pre-hospital deaths in this condition.[12]

Therapeutic advantage

Hospital trials have provided appreciable evidence, concordant with animal experiments, that the benefit of reperfusion by thrombolytic therapy is time-dependent. Data from the Fibrinolytic Therapy Trialists' (FTT) Collaborative Group's overview of nine randomized trials[13] indicated a saving of 35 lives/1,000 when treatment was given within the first two hours, but thrombolysis delayed to between two to four hours reduced this benefit to 25 lives/1,000. The FTT Group suggested a linear reduction in benefit according to time at a rate of 1.6 lives/1,000/hour — but there are theoretical arguments that a linear relationship may not be correct and that the FTT results may underestimate the adverse effect of delays in treatment.[14] The meta-analysis by Boersma *et al*, of 22 randomized thrombolytic trials,[15] supports this view and demonstrated a non-linear benefit/time regression line with a steep initial curve and an important inflection at about two hours (Figure 3b).

Trials of pre-hospital thrombolysis give concordant, if less dramatic, results. The three largest randomized trials comparing pre-hospital with in-hospital thrombolysis — EMIP,[16] MITI[17] and GREAT[18] — demonstrated the feasibility and safety of thrombolysis given in the community. However, through design and practical constraints, these trials were unable to give reliable confirmation that, on an intention-to-treat basis, the mortality at one month post-MI was significantly improved by pre-hospital administration of a thrombolytic agent. A meta-analysis of the the three major trials, with additional data from five smaller studies has, however, shown a significant mortality reduction at 35 days. This was in the context of pre-hospital, compared to in-hospital thrombolysis. In this analysis, the mortality benefit was reduced at a rate of 21/1,000 patients/hour of delay to treatment.[15]

Although a strong case exists for urgent thrombolysis, few studies are available to prove the advantages of reducing the delay in administering other pharmacological agents. Nevertheless, emphasis on the rapid relief of pain and distress with opioids, early use of aspirin and β-blockade in selected patients (particularly those with persistent tachycardia, hypertension or pain) has gained widespread acceptance.[7] The arguments from epidemiology, pathophysiology and therapeutic trials present a persuasive case for providing effective treatment for patients with acute MI as soon as possible after the onset of symptoms. Access to defibrillation, thrombolysis and pain relief should be regarded as urgent, but how far and how quickly can this be achieved in practice before hospital admission?

Practicalities of pre-hospital care

Patient response

The time taken by a patient to summon help varies widely, but usually forms the longest component of the delay to treatment. A recent study from Finland[19] accords well with findings over the past 10 years,[20] although it indicated a relatively short delay time.[21] The median time from the onset of symptoms to calling for help in 1,012 patients treated in hospital for MI was one hour (range: 5–491 min); as many as 21% waited for more than three hours before seeking medical assistance.

The reasons for patient delay are complex and have been explored from both biomedical[22,23] and psychosocial perspectives.[24] The patient's perception and appraisal of symptoms seem to be the most influential factors, although a knowledge of heart symptoms (including the experience of previous angina or MI) appears to exert little effect.[25,26] Factors that have been shown variably to result in a shorter patient delay are age <60, male gender, severity of the infarct and the presence of bystanders (particularly non-relatives).[21,27,28]

Community education campaigns are considered to have had little sustained impact on the behaviour of patients seeking help for cardiac chest pain, even if they have been effective in the short term.[29,30] However this experience should not deter future efforts at public education. Campaigns are likely to be successful if they present information simply with emotional impact and are run persistently over a prolonged period of time. They need also to be based on as much understanding as possible of the individual models of illness and coping that are present in the community.[31]

Role of the professional

General practitioners

When faced with symptoms of acute MI, the majority of patients in the UK still seek professional help from their general practitioner (GP), particularly in rural areas.[32,33] Response times can be rapid, although the overall time from symptoms to the attendance of professional help is usually longer for those patients who summon a GP rather than an ambulance.[32]

A GP can, in principle, administer all essential drug therapy for acute management — opioids, anti-emetics, aspirin, nitrates and thrombolysis. However, in practice, the use of opioids and aspirin appears sub-optimal.[34] Also, although the use of thrombolysis is undoubtedly both feasible and rewarding,[35] substantial hurdles remain before it can be adopted as routine practice.[36] GPs may doubt their ability to interpret an electrocardiogram or otherwise confirm the diagnosis with sufficient confidence to risk the potentially hazardous

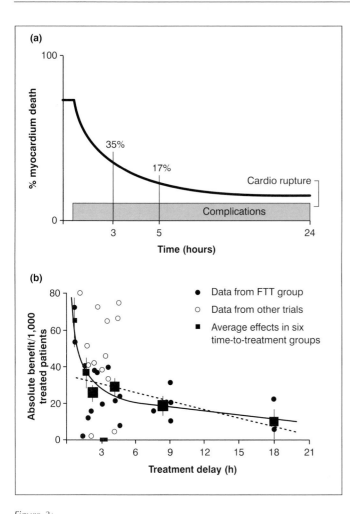

(a)

% myocardium death

100

35%

17%

Cardio rupture

Complications

0

3   5   24

Time (hours)

(b)

Absolute benefit/1,000 treated patients

80

60

40

20

0

● Data from FTT group

○ Data from other trials

■ Average effects in six time-to-treatment groups

3   6   9   12   15   18   21

Treatment delay (h)

Figure 3:
The time-related benefit of reperfusion after coronary occlusion
a) In the experimental model. Redrawn and reproduced with permission[10]
b) From a meta-analysis of 22 randomized trials of thrombolytic therapy. Redrawn and reproduced with permission[7]

effects of giving a thrombolytic agent. In addition, their ability to provide defibrillation as well as effective basic life support — essential ingredients for early care — is by no means uniform across the country. Those with a particular interest and skills in cardiac care provide a high standard of diagnosis and treatment, including resuscitation,[18] but they represent only a minority of practitioners.[36]

Ambulance service

Ambulances staffed by physicians are a feature of many European countries, but, with the exception of Northern Ireland, this is not the case in the UK. They provide a full coronary service, but are expensive. However, ambulances staffed only by paramedics, without a direct medical link, provide highly competent care of the patient with acute MI[17,37,38] and are likely to arrive sooner after the onset of symptoms than a GP.[32] Paramedics are skilled at defibrillation, recording and interpretation of electrocardiograms and insertion of intravenous lines. However, in the UK, their ability to administer drugs for pain relief is limited and their enthusiasm for the use of thrombolysis will remain guarded, at least until the results are available of ongoing trials.

Recommendations

In 1994 a Working Party of the British Heart Foundation published guidelines[39] promoting a dual response from GPs and the ambulance service to fulfil the needs of the patient with acute MI prior to hospital admission. Their recommendations included the goal of achieving both early and adequate pain relief and a call-to-needle time for thrombolysis of ≤90 minutes.

To date there has been little evidence of how far these recommendations have been adopted in practice, or of how variations in organization have been planned to achieve the suggested goals in areas that differ in geography, population and facilities. The public have been encouraged, with variable success, to call an ambulance when there are chest pain symptoms; however, in many cases the GP will still be the first professional summoned,[33] a factor essential for consideration in future service planning.

More recently a Task Force of the European Society of Cardiology and the European Resuscitation Council has announced a series of principal recommendations, divided into basic and optimal, for the care of patients suffering cardiac emergencies (Table 1).[7] Of necessity, these are presented in a general, though helpful, form which is designed for use

Table 1 Principal recommendations on the pre-hospital management of heart attacks[7]

Basic	Optimal
• Widespread knowledge of MI symptoms	• Public media campaigns on coronary symptoms and how to respond
• Access to central emergency number	• Community training in basic life support
• Free calls to ambulance dispatch	• A common European emergency telephone number - 112
• Strategic positioning of ambulances	• Dispatch controlled by physicians
• Use of trained dispatchers and priority-based systems	• Telephone assisted cardio-pulmonary respiration
• All emergency ambulances supplied with efibrillators and electrocardiogram monitors	• Early defibrillation by introducing semi-automatic defibrillators with appropriate training
• All emergency ambulances able to deliver high levels of oxygen	• All emergency ambulances facilitated to record and interpret an electrocardiogram
• Ambulance staff allowed to perform basic life support and defibrillation as in European Resuscitation Council guidelines	• Pre-hospital administration of thrombolysis by a physician, especially when time saved will be more than 60 minutes (strongly recommended)
• Hospital to be notified of the impending arrival of heart attack victims	• Consideration of pre-hospital initiation of thrombolytic therapy by non-physician personnel if any other strategy leads to considerable delays (system under strict medical control)
• Ambulances staffed by two or, preferably, three qualified persons	• Direct admission to coronary care unit or equivalent area for immediate reperfusion therapy
• Registration procedures should not impede triage or delay urgent treatment	

throughout Europe. Unfortunately as a consequence of this they do not embrace the UK concept of the GP. Converting these guidelines into an operational policy for individual localities in each country — a task still required to raise standards of care — will take further work and commitment.

Looking to the future

Two key questions remain: first, how best can we improve the public's reaction to chest pain and, second, who should take the lead both in public education and securing an optimum professional response at local level? This role could be provided from within the ranks of either purchaser or provider, but the essential criteria are strong patient advocacy and a clear understanding of clinical needs. In addition, sensitivity is needed to face the challenges of the primary/secondary care interface, provision of urgent ambulance facilities and good communication. Finally it is essential that this role should capture both the financial resources and authority to implement the changes that are still necessary. All this is needed in order to improve care for patients suffering from MI at the time of greatest risk.

References

1. Bainton CR, Patterson DR. Deaths from coronary heart disease in persons fifty years of age and younger. *N Engl J Med* 1963; **268**: 568–75.
2. Gordon T, Kennel WB. Premature mortality from coronary heart disease. The Framingham Study. *JAMA* 1971; **125**: 1617–25.

3. Kinlen LJ. Incidence and presentation of myocardial infarction in an English Community. *Br Heart J* 1973; **35**: 616–22.

4. Chambless L, Keil U, Dobson A, Mahonen *et al* for the WHO MONICA Project. Population versus clinical view of case fatality from acute coronary heart disease: results from the WHO MONICA Project 1985–1990. *Circulation* 1997; **96**: 3849–59.

5. Sans S, Kesteloot H, Kromhout D on behalf of the Task Force. The burden of cardiovascular mortality in Europe. Task Force of the European Society of Cardiology on Cardiovascular Mortality and Morbidity Statistics in Europe. *Eur Heart J* 1997; **18**: 1231–48.

6. Norris RM on behalf of the United Kingdom Heart Attack Study Collaborative Group. Fatality outside hospital from acute coronary events in three British health districts: 1994–5. *BMJ* 1998; **316**: 1065–70.

7. Task Force of the European Society of Cardiology and Resuscitation. The pre-hospital management of acute heart attacks. *Eur Heart J* 1998; **19**: 1140–64.

8. Davies MJ, Thomas AC. Plaque fissuring: the cause of acute myocardial infarction, sudden ischaemic death and crescendo angina. *Br Heart J* 1985; **53**: 363–73.

9. Poole-Wilson PA. The myocardium in ischaemic heart disease. In: Poole-Wilson PA, Sheridan DJ. *Atherosclerosis in Ischaemic Heart Disease 2: Myocardial Consequenses.* London: Science Press, 1990: 3.1–3.56.

10. Reimer KA, Lowe JE, Rasmussen MM, Jennings RB. The wavefront phenomenon of ischaemic cell death; 1: myocardial infarction size vs duration of coronary occlusion in dogs. *Circulation* 1977; **56**: 786–90.

11. McCance AJ, Thompson, PA Forfar. Increased cardiac sympathetic nervous activity in patients with unstable coronary heart disease. *Eur Heart J* 1993; **14**: 751–7.

12. O`Doherty M, Taylor DI, Quinn E *et al*. Five hundred patients with myocardial infarction monitored within one hour of symptoms. *BMJ* 1983; **286**: 1405–8.

13. Fibrinolytic Therapy Trialists' Collaborative Group. Indications for fibrinolytic therapy in suspected acute myocardial infarction: collaborative overview of early mortality and major morbidity results from all randomised trials of more than 1000 patients. *Lancet* 1994; **343**: 311–22.

14. Rawles J. What is the likely benefit of earlier thrombolysis? *Eur Heart J* 1996; **17**: 991–5.

15. Boersma E, Maas ACP, Deckers JW, Simoons ML. Early thrombolytic treatment in acute myocardial infarction: reappraisal of the golden hour. *Lancet* 1996; **348**: 771–5.

16. The European Myocardial Infarction Project Group. Prehospital thrombolytic therapy in patients with suspected acute myocardial infarction. *N Engl J Med* 1993; **329**: 383–9.

17. Weaver WD, Cerqueira M, Hallstrom AP *et al*. for the Myocardial Infarction Triage and Intervention Project Group: pre-hospital vs hospital-initiated thrombolytic therapy. *JAMA* 1993; **270**: 1211–6.

18. GREAT Group. Feasibility, safety, and efficacy of domiciliary thrombolysis by general practitioners: Grampian region early anistreplase trial. *BMJ* 1992; **305**: 548–53.

19. Hirvonen TPJ, Halinen MO, Kala RA, Olkinuora JT for the Finnish Hospitals` Thrombolysis Survey Group. Delays in thrombolytic therapy for acute myocardial infarction in Finland. *Eur Heart J* 1998; **19**: 885–92.

20. Vincent R. Pre-hospital management. In: Julian D, Braunwald E, eds. *Management of acute myocardial infarction.* London: WB Saunders, 1994: 3–28.

21. Leizorovicz A, Haugh MC, Mercier C, Boissel J-P on behalf of the EMIP Group. Pre-hospital and hospital and hospital delays in thrombolytic treatment in patients with suspected acute myocardial infarction. *Eur Heart J* 1997; **18**: 248–53.

22. Rawles JM, Metcalfe MJ, Shirreffs C *et al*. Association of patient delay with symptoms, cardiac enzymes, and outcome in acute myocardial infarction. *Eur Heart J* 1990; **11**: 643–8.

23. Trent RJ, Rose EL, Adams JN *et al*. Delay between the onset of symptoms of acute myocardial infarction and seeking medical assistance is influenced by left ventricular function at presentation. *Br Heart J* 1995; **73**: 125–8.

24. Dracup K, Moser DK, Eisenberg M *et al*. Causes of delay in seeking treatment for heart attack symptoms. *Soc Sci Med* 1995; **40**: 379–92.

25. Dracup K, Moser DK. Beyond sociodemographics: factors influencing the decision to seek treatment for symptoms of acute myocardial infarction *Heart Lung* 1997; **26**: 253–62.

26. Ruston A, Clayton J, Calnan M. Patients` actions during their cardiac event: qualitative study exploring differences and modifiable factors. *BMJ* 1998; **316**: 1060–5.

27. The GISSI Collaborative Group. Epidemiology of avoidable delay in the care of patients with acute myocardial infarction in Italy. *Arch Intern Med* 1995; **155**: 1481–8.

28. Ottesen MM, Kober L, Jorgensen S, Torp-Pedersen C, on behalf of the TRACE study group. Determinants of delay between symptoms and hospital admission in 5978 patients with acute myocardial infarction. *Eur Heart J* 1996; **17**: 429–37.

29. Rowley JM, Hill JD, Hampton JR, Mitchell JRA. Early reporting of myocardial infarction; impact of an experiment in patient education. *BMJ* 1982; **284**: 1741–6.

30. Herlitz J, Hartford M, Karlson BW *et al*. Effect of a media campaign to reduce delay times for acute for acute myocardial infarction on the burden of chest pain patients in the emergency department. *Cardiology* 1991; **79**: 127–34.

31. Alonzo AA, Reynolds NR. Responding to symptoms and signs of acute myocardial infarction. How do you educate the public? A social-psychologic approach to intervention. *Heart and Lung* 1997; **26**: 263–72.

32. Birkhead JS. Time delays in provision of thrombolytic treatment in six district hospitals. *BMJ* 1992; **305**: 445–8.

33. Rawles JR, Sinclair C, Jennings K *et al*. Call to needle times after acute myocardial infarction in urban and rural areas in northeast Scotland: prospective observational study. *BMJ* 1998; **317**: 576–8.

34. Wyllie HR, Dunn FG. Pre-hospital opiate and aspirin administration in patients with myocardial infarction. *BMJ* 1994; **308**: 760–1.

35. Rawles J. Quantification of the benefit of earlier thrombolytic therapy: 5-year results of the Grampian early anistreplase trial (GREAT). *J Am Coll Cardiol* 1997; **30**: 1181–6.

36. Hannaford P, Vincent R, Ferry S *et al*. Assessment of the practicality and safety of thrombolysis with anistreplase given by general practitioners. *Br J Gen Pract* 1995; **45**: 175–9.

37. Lewis SJ, Holmberg S, Quinn E *et al*. Out-of-hospital resuscitation in East Sussex: 1981–1989. *Br Heart J* 1993; **70**: 568–73.

38. Banerjee S, Rhoden WE. Fast-tracking of myocardial infarction by paramedics. *J Roy Coll Phys* 1998; **32**: 36–8.

39. Weston CFM, Penny WJ, Julian DG, on behalf of the British Heart Foundation Working Group. Guidelines for the early management of patients with myocardial infarction. *BMJ* 1994; **308**: 767–71.

Management of acute myocardial infarction

Anthony Gershlick, University of Leicester & Glenfield Hospital, Leicestershire

Plaque disruption — with the release of intra-plaque content — and activation of coagulation pathways is frequently the initiating event for acute myocardial infarction (MI). Understanding that thrombus formation is central to coronary artery occlusion led to the search for safe and efficient methods of lysing such platelet-rich thrombi and determination of the benefits and limitations of such treatments.

Current therapy

Thrombolytics such as streptokinase and tissue plasminogen activator (tPA) have been shown to improve outcome following MI and, if given sufficiently early (within 12 hours after symptom onset), reduce death rates by about 30% (to ≤10–12%).[1] In reality, however, death rates are higher than in trials, where patient selection tends to occur. Studies have been carried out to compare thrombolytic efficacy in acute MI treatment.[2] tPA appears to have some advantage over streptokinase in younger patients and in those with early presentation after symptoms, anterior infarction and infarction recurrence after previous streptokinase treatment.[3]

Although aspirin has a beneficial effect equivalent to that of thrombolytics, its mode of action is unclear and may not be entirely related to its anticoagulant effects — activity through acetylation of fibrinogen or effects on erythrocyte membrane may play a role.

Administration of angiotensin-converting enzyme (ACE) inhibitors in patients with impaired ventricular function and β-blockers in those with less severely impaired ventricular function improves longer term outcome.[4] Nitrates and prophylactic antiarrythmics do not have any benefit.

Public education to seek help early after the onset of chest pain and improving the speed of thrombolytic delivery through audit review are also important issues in the treatment of acute MI. Performing post-treatment electrocardiograms is uncommon.[5]

Having a patent artery after treatment is important and carries both short- and long-term prognostic benefit. A reperfusion strategy should produce rapid patency. Artery patency may be graded according to Thrombolysis in MI (TIMI) grade (Table 1).[6] The angiographic arm of the Global Utilization of Streptokinase and Tissue Plasminogen Activator for Occluded Coronary Arteries (GUSTO) trial clearly demonstrated that the higher the TIMI grade (ie the more healthy vessel blood flow and luminal narrowing), the lower the mortality at 30 days; patients with TIMI grade 0 (ie complete artery occlusion) at 90 minutes had a 30-day mortality rate of 8.4% while the rate in those with TIMI grade 3 was only 4%.[7] Longer term follow-up from the GUSTO trial patients has recently been reported, demonstrating that establishment of early TIMI grade 3 imparts long term (ie three years) benefits.[8]

Maintaining artery patency is also a very important factor in the treatment of acute MI. The APRICOT trial revealed improved long-term outcome in patients who had maintained artery patency at three months, following its establishment after thrombolytic therapy, compared with those who reoccluded at this time.[9]

Accelerated tPA is currently the most effective thrombolytic available, however, it has been shown to achieve TIMI grade 3 patency in only 50% of patients. Although this is a better result than that of streptokinase, which has been shown to produce grade 3 patency in 30% of

Table 1 Description of coronary artery angiographic images at 90 minutes, and their respective TIMI grades

TIMI Grade	Angiographic image
0	No flow of contrast beyond point of occlusion
1	Penetration with minimal perfusion (contrast fails to opacify entire coronary bed distal to the stenosis for duration of image collection system (cine) run)
2	Partial perfusion (contrast opacifies entire distal coronary but rate of entry and/or clearance is slower in bed of infarct artery than in nearby normally perfused vessel)
3	Complete perfusion (contrast filling and clearance as rapid in infarct vessel as in normally perfused vessels)

patients, much improvement is still required. One reason why tPA is unable to produce better results could be its short half-life, which can cause vessel reocclusion in the first few hours after initial opening. Reocclusion after acute MI occurs in a time-dependent manner with up to 30% of previously open arteries being occluded at three months.[10] Current lytic strategies must therefore be improved, as they do not establish immediate vessel patency in all patients; in addition, a large number of patients are unable to maintain patency.

Improving the outcome post-MI

Since current thrombolytics fail to produce high, early patency rates, the search for new, improved thrombolytics has begun. Safety considerations, particularly the risk of excess bleeding, mean that a therapeutic window needs to be established for any agent under development.

Newer thrombolytics

The ideal thrombolytic must fulfil certain requirements (Table 2). A number of thrombolytics, including mutants or variants of tPA, are currently being developed or undergoing clinical trials. These agents may possess altered resistance to inhibitors such as plasminogen activator inhibitor-1 or require binding to fibrin to become active.[11] Other approaches have involved altering thrombolytic molecules (eg alteration of the kringle 2 region of tPA) to reduce their plasma clearance. Such modifications may improve thrombolytic effectiveness, with increased early patency in most cases (Figure 1).

Reteplase

Reteplase or r-PA is a non-glycosylated deletion mutant of wild type tPA. It differs from tPA at two molecular points with deletion of these molecular domains contributing to its longer half-life.[12] Reteplase is currently being used as an alternative to, but not necessarily an improvement on, tPA.

Lanoteplase and TNK-tPA

Lanoteplase is currently under trial and has been shown to have a particularly high 90 minute patency rate of 75% — this, however, may prove to be a disadvantage if bleeding rates are higher as a consequence. Both lanoteplase and TNK-tPA have longer half-lives as a result of molecular manipulation. It is unlikely that any of the current agents being developed will be dramatically better than tPA and the problems of obtaining very high patency and maintaining it safely will probably be unresolved using modified thrombolytics alone.

Table 2 Requirements of a new thrombolytic

• Non-antigenic	• Plasminogen activator inhibitor-resistant	• Long half-life to allow single bolus administration
• Safe and well-tolerated	• Fibrin-specific	• High and maintained reperfusion rates
		• Cheap

Vampire bat plasminogen activator (bat-PA)

This naturally occurring thrombolytic is similar to human tPA but does not have a plasmin-sensitive processing site. It appears to be resistant to plasminogen activator inhibitor-1 and has greater fibrin selectivity than tPA. Experimental data has shown that bat-PA is efficacious without activating systemic plasminogen and may therefore have a lower bleeding complication rate. Early data suggests very high (>90%) TIMI Grade 3 patency.[13]

Staphylokinase

This is a protein produced by *Staphylococcus aureus* that has profibrinolytic properties. A recombinant form, staphylokinase recombinant (STAR) was found to be less immunogenic and more active against platelet-rich, arterial clots than streptokinase. This has now been evaluated in small clinical trials with 10–20 mg of STAR given over 30 minutes producing similar coronary recanalization rates to accelerated tPA, but without any fibrinogen breakdown (ie significantly more fibrin-specificity than tPA). Unfortunately all patients developed STAR-neutralizing antibodies from the second week after treatment, suggesting that this agent may not be as hypoallergenic as originally hoped.

Any new strategy, regimen or agent must be tested against current therapies, proceeding towards clinical trials that will require substantial numbers of patients to show a mortality difference.

Anti-thrombins

Up to 30% of patients experience artery reocclusion three months after successful thrombolysis.[14] Heparin is the mainstay of treatment when tPA is used. Although heparin is relatively safe, it has a number of disadvantages: it requires endogenous co-factors for activity (principally anti-thrombin III and heparin co-factor II); it is inactive against fibrin-bound thrombin and is unable to displace thrombin bound to platelets; and its action can be neutralized by products released by activated platelets (eg platelet factor 4).

As a result, new, direct-acting anti-thrombins such as hirudin, argatroban and efegatran have been developed. Although all are anti-thrombin III independent, their precise mechanism of inhibition varies. The latter two agents act as reversible inhibitors. Hirudin binds to both the active catalytic and substrate recognition sites of thrombin and inhibits thrombin-catalyzed activation of factors V, VIII and XIII and thrombin-induced platelet activation. Hirudin has been shown to prevent rethrombosis after tPA administration in animals.[15]

Three large clinical trials with Hirudin commenced in 1994 but were discontinued as a result of excess intracerebral bleeding.

Preliminary results from the GUSTO IIb study suggested no increase in clinical benefit with hirudin use at a lower dose.[16] The narrow therapeutic window for these new anti-thrombins make it difficult at present to define their exact role in clinical practice.

Figure 1: TIMI grade 3 patency rates for some of the newer thrombolytics compared with established agents

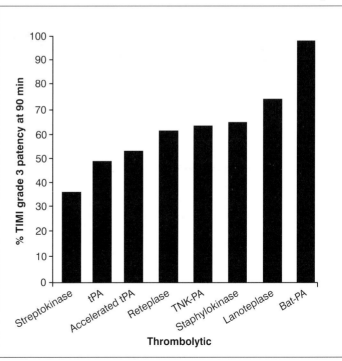

New antiplatelet treatments

Platelets are responsible for thrombus generation following arterial injury. Studies by Collen revolutionized our understanding of effective antiplatelet therapy,[17] clarifying the major role of the fibrinogen receptor (glycoprotein IIb/IIIa) on platelets in platelet-platelet aggregation and fibrin-platelet development progressing to a mature thrombus. As aspirin only influences one activation pathway in platelets, it is unable to solely inhibit the stimulatory effects of high doses of collagen and thrombin on platelets.

A more effective antiplatelet therapy is one that inhibits the pathway that activates glycoprotein IIb/IIIa. A humanized monoclonal antibody (7E3) against this receptor is available and has been shown to improve artery patency in animals when administered alone.[18] Platelet inhibition, low bleeding rates and low incidence of recurrent ischaemia were reported when 7E3 was used after tPA.

Synthetic derivatives of glycoprotein IIb/IIIa receptor inhibitors are also available. These have been tested extensively in patients with acute coronary syndromes and those undergoing high and lower risk coronary intervention. Early benefit is seen but not always maintained.[19]

One example of a glycoprotein IIb/IIIa receptor inhibitor is Tirofiban. The PRISM-PLUS trial investigated the effects of Tirofiban plus unfractionated herapin in 1,915 patients with unstable angina or non-Q wave MI. The composite end-point of death, MI or refractory ischaemia at seven days was shown to be reduced by 32%; the risk of MI at seven days was reduced by 47%.[20] Tirofiban is currently undergoing regulatory approval and is expected to be launched this year. Another receptor inhibitor under trial is Eptifibatide, which showed similar results.[21] Table 3 summarizes and compares the efficacy and pharmacokinetics of both drugs.

Oral agents such as Xemilofiban and Lamifiban are currently under trial and it is expected that they will be used in patients with coronary disease. Studies have shown that combining these powerful antiplatelet agents with thrombolytics may be safe and produce high patency rates despite a 50% thrombolytic dose reduction. The early pilot results using synthetic integrelin in acute MI patients are also encouraging suggesting that an improvement in coronary artery patency and reduction in recurrent ischaemic events may be possible.

GUSTO-IV will test 7E3 as adjunctive therapy to reteplase. Such studies will not be designed to replace aspirin but will determine whether or not the action of additional antiplatelet therapy through alternative pathways has added advantages. Bleeding complications will need to be carefully assessed. Of the various therapeutic options that might be considered as adjunctive to thrombolysis, these powerful platelet receptor inhibitors appear to have true potential.

Primary angioplasty

This is an alternative therapy to thrombolysis in acute MI. It involves the use of an intracoronary wire and balloon to mechanically remove the thrombus and dilate the underlying stenotic lesion; patients must be taken to a catheter laboratory as expeditiously as possible.

Angioplasty produces patency rates of 99% with 96% being TIMI 3, much higher than the current best rate of 54% TIMI 3 flow with thrombolysis (Figure 2).[22,23] In the Zwolle study, 90% of patients achieved TIMI 3 flow with angioplasty while only 55% did in the streptokinase group.[24] The study revealed that angioplasty was associated with a lower enzyme rise, better left ventricular function, less reinfarction (7% v 30%) and lower 31 month mortality (5% v 13%, $p=0.03$). The longer term, event-free survival (ie no MI, cardiac death or need for reintervention)

Table 3 Key characteristics of Tirofiban[20] and Eptifibatide[21]

Glycoprotein IIb/IIIa receptor inhibitor	Risk reduction in primary end-point at seven days (%)	Risk reduction in primary end-point at 30 days (%)	Platelet-bound half-life
Tirofiban	5	3.5	Short
Eptifibatide	1.5	1.5	Short

has been shown by some authors to favour angioplasty while other meta-analysed data is less convincing about the longer term benefit although this included some trials with very small numbers resulting in wide confidence intervals. Pooling of the data suggests that high-risk patients (older age, larger infarcts and anterior infarcts) in particular benefit both in terms of mortality and reinfarction. There is evidence that outcome is dependent on volume of angioplasties performed. A cost benefit analysis carried out in Europe and the US indicated that primary percutaneous transluminal coronary angioplasty is not as expensive as thrombolysis in the longer term.

More recently in the GUSTO II trial, the direct angioplasty arm failed to show significant benefits compared to tPA (death, reinfarction, disabling strokes 10% v 13%, $p=0.06$). This may be related to a lower achieved TIMI grade 3 patency in this study compared to previous studies (74% v >90%). Angioplasty for acute MI has

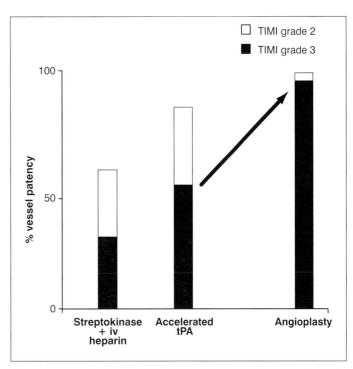

Figure 2: Use of balloon angioplasty in treating acute MI compared with currently best available thrombolytics

to be good, and may need to involve deployment of stents and the use of glycoprotein IIb/IIIa receptor blockers. Knowing the state of the coronary artery may allow for better subsequent management of patients, including shorter hospital stays.

There are, however, problems related to limited resources of angioplasty for acute MI in terms of personnel and finance. Most patients in the UK are admitted to units without invasive facilities and current resources allow for only about 17,000 angioplasties per year, concentrated in approximately 54 units.

The value of primary angioplasty over thrombolysis has not yet been definitively established. If it is to be undertaken, however, it must be performed by experienced operators who are more likely to achieve the TIMI Grade 3 required for acute and longer term advantage. It is most probable that primary angioplasty will not become established practice in the UK – patients currently considered as definite candidates for angioplasty (contraindications to thrombolysis, cardiogenic shock and failure to reperfuse after thrombolysis) must be clearly identified and can be transferred for primary angioplasty if necessary .

Optimizing reperfusion therapies

Primary angioplasty is safe but impractical. Combining the strategies of primary thrombolytic with adjunctive therapy and angioplasty for those with failed thrombolysis may become the optimal therapy. Selecting patients whose arteries remain occluded after thrombolysis has been shown to be feasible with a high sensitivity and specificity.[25,26] In the DANAMI trial, patients shown to have reversible ischaemia within two weeks of thrombolytic therapy and who were randomized to intervention had better recurrent ischaemia results than those treated conservatively.[27] After 24 hours post-thrombolytic administration, however, myocardial salvage of those with occluded arteries becomes a case of providing benefit to those patients who, because of collaterals, will select themselves out for benefit. In the British Heart Foundation-funded REACT trial, patients will be assessed for patency at 90 minutes after thrombolytic administration on the basis of ECGs. Those assessed as having an occluded artery will be randomized to either conservative treatment, further thrombolytic or intervention. This study will involve 1,200 patients and will be based in the UK.

Conclusion

Thrombolytic therapy with adjunctive aspirin has significantly improved mortality following MI. Public education about the need to recognize the implications of chest pain, particularly in those with risk factors for coronary disease, is imperative to reduce the delay to thrombolysis. Vessel patency must also be optimized as this correlates with early and longer term survival.

New thrombolytics are becoming available and may improve patency, but they will need to be tested against current therapies. Trials of new anti-thrombins for reducing vessel reocclusion have demonstrated a narrow therapeutic window for these agents — their future role remains unclear. Potent platelet inhibitors are more likely to lead to higher rates of immediate and sustained vessel patency; oral formulations may soon be commercially available. Primary angioplasty could prove to be the definitive treatment in selected cases, provided the procedure is undertaken early enough to be of benefit. Limited resources may be the inhibiting factor in widespread use of this treatment therapy. A combination of drug-based thrombolysis and coronary intervention for those who fail to perfuse could be the best way forward.

References

1. ISIS-2 Collaborative Group. Randomised trial of intravenous streptokinase, oral aspirin, both or neither among 17,187 cases of suspected acute myocardial infarction. *Lancet* 1988; **2**: 349–60.

2. ISIS-3. A randomised comparison of streptokinase vs tissue plasminogen activator vs anistreplase and of aspirin plus heparin vs aspirin along among 41,299 cases of suspected acute myocardial infarction. ISIS-3 (Third International Study of Infarct Survival) Collaborative Group (see comments). *Lancet* 1992; **339**: 753–70.

3. Tung CY, Granger CB, Sloan MA *et al*. Effects of stroke on medical resource use and costs in acute myocardial infarction. GUSTO I investigators. Global utilisation of streptokinase and tissue plasminogen activator for occluded coronary arteries study. *Circulation* 1999; **99**(3): 370–6.

4. ISIS-4. A randomised trial comparing oral captopril versus placebo, oral mononitrate versus placebo, and intravenous magnesium sulphate versus control among 58,043 patients with suspected acute myocardial infarction. *Lancet* 1995; **345**: 669–85.

5. Prendagast BD, Shandell A, Buchalter MB. What do we do when thrombolysis fails? *Int J Cardiol* 1997; **61**: 39–42.

6. Puma JA, Sketch MH Jr, Thompson TD *et al*. Support for the open-artery hypothesis in survivors of acute myocardial infarction: analysis of 11,228 patients treated with thrombolytic therapy. *Am J Cardiol* 1999; **83**(4): 482–7.

7. The GUSTO Angiographic Investigators. The effects of tissue plasminogen activator, streptokinase, or both on coronary patency, ventricular function, and survival after acute myocardial infarction. *N Engl J Med* 1993; **329**:1615–22.

8. Ross AM, Coyne KS, Moreyra E *et al*. Extended mortality benefit of early postinfarction. GUSTO-I Angiographic Investigators. Global Utilization of Streptokinase and Tissue Plaminogen Activator for Occluded Coronary Arteries Trial. *Circulation* 1998; **97**: 1549–56.

9. Brouwer MA, Bohncke JR, Veen G *et al*. Adverse long-term effects of reocclusion after coronary thrombolysis. *J Am Coll Cardiol* 1995; **26**: 1440–4.

10. Meijer A, Verheugt FW, Werter CJ *et al*. Aspirin versus coumadin in the prevention of reocclusion and recurrent ischaema after successful thrombolysis: a prospective placebo-controlled angiographic study. Results of the APRICOT Study. *Circulation* 1993; **87**(5): 1524–30.

11. Verstraete M, Lijnen HR, Collen D. Thrombolytic agents in development. *Drugs* 1995; **50**(1): 29–42.

12. Martin U, Kohler J, Sponer G *et al*. Pharmacokinetics of the novel recombinant plasminogen activator BM 06.022 in rats, dogs, and non-human primates. *Fibrinolysis* 1992; **6**: 39–43.

13. Mellott MJ, Stabilito II, Holahan MA *et al*. Vampire bat salivary plasminogen activator promotes rapid and sustained reperfusion without concomitant system plasminogen activation in a canine model of arterial thrombosis. *Arterioscler Thromb Vasc Biol* 1992; **12**(2): 212–21.

14. Brouwer MA, Bohneke JR, Veen G *et al*. Adverse long-term effects of reocclusion after coronary thrombolysis. *J Am Coll Cardiol* 1995; **26**(6): 1440–4.

15. Electricwala A, Atkinson T. Effect of hirudin on tissue plasminogen activator-induced clot lysis. *Blood Coagul Fibrinolysis* 1990; **1**(3): 267–71.

16. Antman EM, Braunwald E. Trials and tribulations of thrombin inhibition. *Eur Heart J* 1996; **17**: 971–3.

17. Kohmura C, Gold HK, Yasuda T *et al*. A chimeric murine/human antibody Fab fragment directed against the platelet GP IIb/IIIa receptor enhances and sustains arterial thrombolysis with recombinant tissue-type plasminogen activator in baboons. *Arterioscler Thromb Vasc Biol* 1993; **13**(12): 1837–42.

18. Gold H, Cigarroa JE, Ferrell MA *et al*. Enhanced endogenous coronary thrombolysis during acute myocardial following selective platelet receptor blockade with ReoPro. Presented at the 69th Scientific session at the American heart Association Meeting Nov 1996.

19. Adgey AA. An overview of the results of clinical trials with glycoprotein IIb/IIIa inhibitors. *Eur Heart J* 1998; **19**(suppl D): D10–21.

20. PRISM–PLUS Study Investigators. Inhibition of the platelet glycoprotein IIb/IIIa receptor with Tirofiban in unstable angina and non-Q wave myocardial infarction. *N Engl J Med* 1998; **338**: 1488–97.

21. PURSUIT Trial Investigators. Inhibition of glycoprotein IIb/IIIa with Eptifibatide in patients with acute coronary syndromes. *N Engl J Med* 1998; **339**: 436–43.

22. O'Neill WW, Brodie BR, Ivanhoe R. Primary coronary angioplasty for acute myocardial infarction (the Primary Angioplasty Registry). *Am J Cardiol* 1994; **73**(9): 627–34.

23. Nunn CM, O'Neill WW, Rothbaum D *et al*. Long-term outcome after primary angioplasty: report from the primary angioplasty in myocardial infarction (PAMI-I) trial. *J Am Coll Cardiol* 1999; **33**(3): 640–6.

24. Vant Hof AW, Liem A, Suryapranata H *et al*. Angiographic assessment of myocardial reperfusion in patients treated with primary angioplasty for acute myocardial infarction: myocardial blush grade. *Circulation* 1998; **97**(23): 2302–6.

25. Klootwijk P, Langer A, Meij S *et al*. Non-invasive prediction of reperfusion and coronary artery patency by continuous ST segment monitoring in the GUSTO-I trial. *Eur Heart J* 1996; **17**(5): 689–98.

26. Buszman P, Szafranek A, Kalarus Z, Gasior M. Use of changes in ST segment elevation for prediction of infarct artery recanalisation in acute myocardial infarction. *Euro Heart J* 1995; **16**(9): 1207–14.

27. Madsen JK, Grande P, Saunamaki K *et al*. Danish multicenter randomised study of invasive versus conservative treatment in patients with ischaemia after thrombolysis in acute myocardial infarction (DANAMI) *Circ* 1997; **96**: 748–55.

Hospital investigation

Keith Fox, Cardiovascular Research Unit, The Royal Infirmary of Edinburgh, Edinburgh

The major treatment strategies in acute myocardial infarction (MI) are based on large-scale clinical trial data and the evolution of international, national and local guidelines.[1] There are consequently clear strategies for basic and advanced life support following cardiac arrest and for the management of arrhythmias, reperfusion (principally by thrombolysis) and adjunctive treatment to limit myocardial damage. During the early recovery phase there are now extensive data to support specific treatments in heart failure and the initiation of secondary prevention strategies.[2] Given such evidence, it is important to consider which patients should be investigated, how they should be investigated and when.

Rationale for further investigations in acute MI

For every thousand patients who sustain an acute MI, about 180 die within the first hour and a further 180 within the following 24 hours.[3] The Multicentre Post-infarction Research Group demonstrated that, for those patients who survive the acute phase of MI, one-year mortality averages about 10% and three-year mortality about 15-25%.[4] The 10-year mortality cumulatively reaches almost 50%.[5,6] However, these averaged figures obscure substantial differences in risk for various categories of patients.

Multivariate analysis has demonstrated that the factors which independently predict a higher risk of mortality are age, congestive heart failure, previous MI and diabetes mellitus. A number of other factors may be contributory — such as the impact of recurrent or persistent ischaemia, or the development of specific arrhythmias — but these have not yet emerged as independent predictors in multivariate analysis. There is evidence to support the use of such variables in determining risk.

Overall, the rational basis for investigation in patients following hospitalization for acute MI focuses upon the identification of those individuals that are at higher risk and for whom specific interventions or treatments may provide improved outcome.

Risk stratification

Clinically, a patient can frequently be identified as high-risk or low-risk, based on a combination of clinical features and complicating events. Clinically, however, a systematic approach to risk stratification is seldom applied, yet such an approach may reveal higher risk patients among those that appear clinically uncomplicated.

Among pre-existing risk factors, age and previous MI are the most important. In contrast, complicating events — such as heart failure, recurrent arrhythmias and mechanical complications or provoked ischaemia — are indicative of the severity of underlying ischaemia or infarction. Although the rise in cardiac enzymes can provide a rough indication of the severity of myocardial damage, it is often misleading. First, infrequent sampling may miss the peak in cardiac enzymes, plus the 'area under the curve' is more predictive of the extent of damage than the peak itself. Second, reperfusion produces an abrupt release of enzymes with a higher peak but a narrower curve. In addition, the sequence of cardiac enzymes may only be available retrospectively.

Heart failure requires specific mention. From multivariate analyses it is one of the most powerful independent predictors of a poor prognosis following MI. More than 30% of patients with overt heart failure (New York Heart Association Classification III or IV) die within one year.[7] Furthermore, trials of angiotensin-converting enzyme (ACE) inhibitor therapy demonstrate improvement in survival among patients with overt or significant asymptomatic left ventricular

21

dysfunction (LVD) (ejection fraction <40%). With appropriate doses of angiotensin receptor antagonists, similar findings may apply and the two agents may be synergistic. In the Survival and Ventricular Enlargement trial (SAVE) trial,[8] mortality was 25% in the placebo group and 20% in a group randomized to captopril (started three to 16 days after infarction) over a median follow-up of 3.5 years. Recently presented data from the CIBIS 2 and MERIT trials demonstrate important benefits for β-blockers in ambulant patients with heart failure. These figures illustrate the profound influence and extent of myocardial damage and consequent heart failure upon survival.

High-risk patients

High risk may be determined by the combination of pre-existing risk factors, the development of complications of the infarction or evidence that a large volume of myocardium is at risk of recurrent ischaemia (Table 1).

Medium-risk patients

Such patients may have less severe pre-existing clinical features and only moderate or transient heart failure. Ischaemia may be precipitated by exertion, rather than spontaneously or at rest (Table 2).

Low-risk patients

In contrast, low-risk patients are free of both prior risk factors and complicating events. The exclusion characteristics of certain clinical trials may lead to predominantly low-risk patients being included and the false impression that the mortality from MI is lower than exists in reality (Table 3).

Investigations

Left ventricular function and heart failure

Patients that present with acute pulmonary oedema or other features of overt heart failure are already in the high-risk category. Echocardiography may be useful to assess ventricular function in the remaining, apparently unaffected, segments of myocardium and also to detect papillary muscle dysfunction, ventricular septal defects and evidence of pre-existing cardiac dilatation or hypertrophy.

Echocardiography is particularly useful among patients with transient features of heart failure. A comparison between an earlier examination during the features of heart failure and a repeat examination in the recovery phase may provide the best estimate of the severity of myocardial damage (and how much may be transiently impaired or 'stunned'). Where available, stress echo provides a more accurate prediction of a potentially viable myocardium. Among low-risk patients, echocardiography can be restricted to the recovery phase, in order to detect asymptomatic LVD and, consequently, the need for ACE inhibitor treatment.

Arrhythmias

Continuous electrocardiographic monitoring with automated systems allows the detection of arrhythmias based on changes in heart rate or electrocardiogram (ECG) morphology.

Table 1 High-risk patients

Pre-existing clinical features and complicating events:	
• Age >65 years	• Acute mechanical complications (ventricular septal defect, papillary muscle rupture)
• Multiple risk factors (eg hypertension, diabetes)	• Angina at rest or on minimal exertion
• Previous myocardial infarction and impaired left ventricular function	• Recurrent arrhythmias
• Persistent heart failure or shock	• Unable to perform an exercise tolerance test
• Severely impaired ventricular function	

Table 2 Medium-risk patients

Pre-existing clinical features and complicating events:

- Age 55–65 years
- Diabetes mellitus
- Previous myocardial infarction

- Transient heart failure
- Impaired ventricular function (moderate)
- Angina or ischaemia precipitated by exertion

Table 3 Low-risk patients

Pre-existing clinical features and complicating events:

- Age <55 years
- No previous myocardial infarction
- No previous heart failure
- No previous major risk factors (hypertension, diabetes)

- Event-free clinical course
- No ischaemia or angina on exercise testing or other forms of stress testing
- No evidence of heart failure

However, a full 12-lead ECG should be obtained urgently following the development of an arrhythmia (unless emergency resuscitation is necessary) in order to differentiate the site and mode of conduction of various arrhythmias (for example distinguishing supraventricular from ventricular, tachycardia and revealing occult re-entrant arrhythmias).

Ventricular tachycardia or ventricular fibrillation occurring during the acute ischaemic phase of MI (for example the first 24 hours) does not carry a sinister long-term prognosis, provided that the acute event is treated promptly. However, where ventricular tachycardia or ventricular fibrillation have caused collapse (and in the absence of precipitating acute ischaemia) further investigations are necessary. Such patients are at potential risk of recurrent arrhythmias.

Depending upon the extent of prior myocardial damage or the underlying condition, cardiac catheterization and electrophysiological testing may be required. Cardiac catheterization can reveal the extent of underlying coronary artery disease (or its absence) and electrophysiological testing can reveal the source and significance of specific arrhythmias. Such testing usually requires investigation in specialized centres. In some patients the arrhythmia may be provoked or revealed on ambulatory monitoring or exercise tolerance testing. Recent studies of implantable defibrillators (for example the MADIT trial)[9] have revealed a 50–75% reduction in the risk of arrhythmic deaths with such treatment.

Coronary angiography

Although coronary angiography is routinely performed following MI in some countries and healthcare systems, this strategy has not been validated in large scale clinical trials. Indeed, previous trials have shown that late angiography following thrombolysis does not necessarily result in improved outcome. However, angiography is clearly indicated for patients with spontaneous or provoked ischaemia in the early post-MI phase. Where ischaemia is provoked on minimal exertion or mobilization of the patient, the optimal strategy would be to undertake angiography before hospital discharge. Where the evidence of ischaemia is provoked at a high work-load then such investigations could be deferred and performed electively on an outpatient basis (provided there are no other markers of higher risk).

Coronary angiography should be undertaken in the early post-infarction period when there is:

- angina/ischaemia that does not respond to pharmacological therapy
- angina or evidence of myocardial ischaemia at rest
- exercise or other stress-induced angina or myocardial ischaemia at a lower work load, or on holter monitoring or when there has been little or no increase in heart rate.

Coronary angiography should be considered when there is:

- angina, or objective evidence of provokable myocardial ischaemia (in the absence of features described above)

- post-infarction angina that is not responding to pharmacological therapy
- severe LVD
- complex ventricular arrhythmias more than 48 hours post-MI. Revascularization may be required on prognostic grounds — when there are significant two-vessel or three-vessel disease, especially when ventricular function is impaired — or to relieve symptoms of ischaemia.

Current evidence suggests that angioplasty and coronary bypass surgery have slightly different roles post-MI. Surgical revascularization is recommended for patients with left main coronary artery disease or three-vessel coronary artery disease and impaired left ventricular function (or other indications for revascularization). Angioplasty is indicated for patients who have one- or two- vessel disease and also lesions suitable for the technique (with or without stent implantation). Large-scale trials suggest that angioplasty has a similar mortality outcome, in the longer term, to surgery, but that it results in reduced symptom relief and a greater need for repeat procedures. However, more modern angioplasty and stent implantation may have an improved outcome, with a reduced need for repeat procedures. Angioplasty is initially cheaper than surgery, less invasive and requires shorter hospitalization.

Unstable angina post-MI

Patients with unstable angina following acute MI are at high risk. An episode of unstable angina within five days of infarction is associated with a one-year mortality rate of more than 20%. A Danish multi-centre randomized study (the DANAMI study) investigated angiography followed by angioplasty or coronary bypass surgery, versus a conservative strategy following thrombolysis among 1,108 patients aged below 70.[10] It identified patients with symptomatic ischaemia or ischaemia provoked by exercise testing without symptoms. After two and a half years the aggressive strategy had produced a significant reduction in the combined endpoint of death, non-fatal MI and unstable angina without hospitalization.

There is consequently support for the concept of performing revascularization in patients with spontaneous or provoked ischaemia. However, there is no evidence to support a generalized strategy for routine angiography and revascularization following MI. Routine angiography is frequently justified on the basis of the prognostic information provided (the extent of underlying coronary artery disease is a strong predictor of subsequent outcome). However, among patients without readily provoked ischaemia, the evidence to support revascularization of incidentally-detected lesions is lacking.

Stress testing

The most widely performed stress testing is electrocardiographic exercise testing, the timing of which has been a matter of controversy. Optimally, a pre-discharge exercise tolerance test may reveal occult but readily provoked ischaemia or arrhythmias and may therefore indicate the need for more invasive investigations and specific treatments. Deferring such stress testing until the time of outpatient review may allow more patients to complete higher levels of exercise, but there may be risks during the interval among those with readily provoked ischaemia or arrhythmias. Recent studies have demonstrated that a symptom-limited stress test can be performed before hospital discharge (to reveal readily provoked ischaemia and arrhythmias) with a very low risk of complications.[10]

Stress echocardiography is more sensitive and specific but requires high levels of technical expertise to produce consistent and reliable results. Pharmacological stress and nuclear perfusion scanning — for example stress thallium or sestamibi — imaging is again more sensitive and specific than exercise ECG, with sensitivities and specificities similar to stress echo performed in expert hands. The nuclear imaging techniques are reliable and reproducible in experienced centres but they do expose patients to an additional radiation burden.

Inability to perform an exercise test is also a predictor of an adverse outcome. Data from the GISSI-2 study indicate a threefold increase in the risk of reinfarction among such patients.[11] Overall, the risk of recurrent non-fatal reinfarction in MI survivors is increased 1.7-

fold as a result of previous MI and 1.5-fold as a result of angina post-MI. However, it is important to remember that almost 50% of reinfarctions occur in patients without commonly identified risk factors.

Invasive haemodynamic monitoring

The insertion of a balloon tipped catheter via a vein to the right heart and pulmonary artery allows measurement of filling pressures of the left heart, 'the pulmonary wedge pressure' and, when combined with a thermistor, can determine cardiac output. Such catheters are particularly useful in patients with severe haemodynamic compromise, where regular measurement of cardiac output and pressures allows the titration of inotropic support and the maintenance of optimal fluid balance. In the context of acute MI such techniques should only be performed in experienced hands and in appropriately equipped CCUs or Intensive Care Units.

Computed tomography and magnetic resonance imaging scanning

The improved resolution associated with modern computed tomography (CT) and magnetic resonance imaging (MRI) imaging devices allows the detection and localization of acute aortic dissections, aneurysms and a number of other disorders of the mediastinum and great vessels. Such techniques can also reveal pericardial effusions, myocardial thickness and calcification. In the future, experimental MRI perfusion imaging may allow regular clinical assessment of regional myocardial perfusion.

Secondary prevention strategies

The long-term benefits associated with secondary prevention strategies mandate that all potentially eligible patients receive such treatment. Most of the secondary prevention strategies do not require specific investigations for implementation. Smoking cessation, for example, prevents 15 deaths and 45 reinfarctions per 1,000 patient treatment years; aspirin therapy prevents seven deaths, nine non-fatal MIs and nine non-fatal strokes and statins (HMG-CoA reductase inhibitors) result in approximately seven fewer deaths, 11 revascularizations, 12 non-fatal MIs, three fewer strokes and four fewer heart failure patients, per 1,000 patient treatment years.[2] Evidence also supports the use of β-blocker therapy post-MI. Detailed discussions of secondary prevention strategies are beyond the scope of this review but are included in subsequent chapters.

Conclusion

The combination of clinical assessment and readily available investigations can provide a reliable basis for risk stratification among post-MI patients. Risk assessment now forms part of the subconscious evaluation of each patient among experienced clinicians, but a more systematic and thorough approach is indicated.

The investigations required post-MI are designed to detect impaired ventricular function, arrhythmias, mechanical complications of infarction and readily provoked ischaemia. Biochemical and haematological blood tests are also part of the routine assessment of patients during and following MI. Thus, the investigation strategy is based on a targeted approach which aims to stratify risk and identify those major complications which are amenable to treatment. Such a strategy is not only rational, but potentially cost-effective.

References

1. Task force on the management of acute myocardial infarction, the European Society of Cardiology. European Society of Cardiology Guidelines. Acute myocardial infarction: pre-hospital and in-hospital management. *Eur Heart J* 1996; **17**: 43–63.
2. Sivers F. Evidence-based strategies for secondary prevention of coronary heart disease. London: Science Press, 1996.
3. Fox KAA. Management of patients following myocardial infarction. *Medicine* 1997; **25**: 68–72.

4. Dwyer EM Jr, McMaster P, Greenberg H, Multicentre Postinfarction Research Group. Nonfatal cardiac events and recurrent infarction in the year after acute myocardial infarction. *J Am Coll Cardiol* 1984; **4**: 695–702.

5. Herlitz J, Karlson BW, Hjalmarson A. Ten-year mortality rate after development of acute myocardial infarction in relation to clinical history and observations during hospital stay: Experience from the Goteborg metoprolol trial. *Coronary Artery Disease* 1993; **4**(12): 1077–83.

6. Franzosi MG, Santoro E, De Vita C *et al*. Ten-year follow-up of the first megatrial testing thrombolytic therapy in patients with acute myocardial infarction. *Circulation* 1998; **98**: 2659–65.

7. The SOLVD Investigators. Effect of enalapril on survival in patients with reduced left ventricular ejection fractions and congestive heart failure. *N Engl J Med* 1991; **325**: 293–302.

8. Pfeffer MA, Brauwald E, Moye LA *et al* (on behalf of the SAVE Investigators). Effect of captopril on mortality and morbidity in patients with left ventricular dysfunction after myocardial infarction: results of the Survival and Ventricular Enlargement Trial. *N Engl J Med* 1992; **327**: 669–77.

9. Moss AJ, Hall WJ, Cannons DS *et al*. Improved survival with an implanted defibrillator in patients with coronary disease at high risk for ventricular arrhythmia. *N Engl J Med* 1996; **335**: 1933–40.

10. Madsen JK, Grande P, Saunamaki K *et al*. Danish multicentre randomised study of invasive *versus* conservative treatment in patients with inducible ischaemia after thrombolysis in acute myocardial infarction (DANAMI). *Circulation* 1997; **96**: 748–55.

11. Volpi A, De Vita C, Franzosi MG *et al*. Determinants of 6-month mortality in survivors of myocardial infarction after thrombolysis. Results of the GISSI-2 data base. *Circulation* 1993; **88**: 416–29.

Community investigation

Manish Gandhi, Wessex Cardiothoracic Centre, Southampton University Hospital, Southampton

The purpose of investigating myocardial infarction (MI) patients in the community is ultimately to improve their quality of life and prognosis. MI patients in the community fall into two categories — patients at risk of impending MI and patients who have been discharged from hospital following MI. This paper will focus first, on the investigation of post-MI patients in the community and, second, on the importance of identifying patients at risk of MI and the impact of this strategy on the reduction of overall MI mortality.

Figure 1 illustrates the importance of the two patient categories. Post-MI patients in the community represent only 40% of acute MI survivors. Recent data show that 50% of patients with acute MI die within one month of their infarct and two-thirds of these deaths occur before reaching hospital.[1] It is immediately apparent, therefore, that hospital interventions, such as thrombolysis or coronary angioplasty, have a very limited impact on reducing overall mortality from acute MI. Interventions targeted at patients in the community are likely to have a much larger impact on improving survival.

Post-infarction patients

Patients discharged from hospital to the care of their general practitioner (GP) following MI may be regarded as being at a low risk of further cardiovascular events, at least in the short term. Most have had risk stratification with non-invasive investigations, such as exercise testing; those with recurrent symptoms and low workload positive exercise tests have undergone coronary revascularization. Nevertheless, patients who have had a previous MI within the community have a six-fold higher rate of cardiovascular events compared with healthy subjects.

A clear indication for initiating investigation is the occurrence of new symptoms. Angina, dyspnoea and palpitation are the most frequently reported symptoms and relate to epicardial coronary artery disease, an infarcted myocardium as a failing pump, and as a substrate for arrhythmias, respectively. Recent advances in therapeutic interventions allow reductions in both the morbidity and mortality associated with these symptoms.

Recurrent angina

A patient in the community presenting with angina following MI should have an exercise test for two important reasons: first, to provide an objective measure of

Figure 1:
Outcome of myocardial infarction in the community and hospital.
Redrawn and reproduced with permission[1]

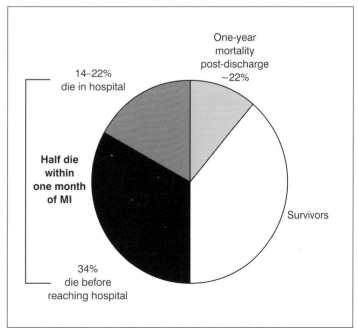

One-year mortality post-discharge ~22%

14–22% die in hospital

Half die within one month of MI

Survivors

34% die before reaching hospital

the patient's functional limitation and second, to identify patients with a low workload who have the most to gain from coronary revascularization.

Most trials comparing medical therapy with either percutaneous transluminal coronary angioplasty (PTCA) or coronary artery bypass surgery (CABG) are outdated because of rapid advances in revascularization techniques. Some of the original conclusions, however, do still hold true. CABG is more effective than medical therapy in relieving angina in the short and medium term, but this advantage diminishes over time with increasing graft re-occlusion. About one-third of patients require repeat CABG after ten years. The magnitude of survival benefit of CABG over medical therapy also diminishes over time, for example from 39% at five years to 17% at 10 years. It is of most use for patients with three-vessel disease, especially in the presence of impaired left ventricular function.[2]

Very few trials have compared medical therapy with coronary angioplasty. Limited data suggest that, for patients with single vessel disease, angioplasty offers better relief from angina in the short term, with no difference in survival.[2] Compared with coronary angioplasty, bypass surgery offers more effective relief from angina after one year with no significant difference in the rate of either MI or death, but this advantage diminishes with time. Observational data suggests that the benefit to risk ratio favours PTCA over CABG in less severe disease.[2]

The advent of intra-coronary stenting requires complete re-evaluation of the relative benefits of the revascularization strategies compared with medical therapy. Elective intra-coronary stenting as an adjunct to balloon angioplasty reduces the rate of restenosis, and therefore the need for repeat intervention, from about 20–35% to 10% during the first year.[3] The deployment of stents also reduces abrupt vessel closure during the procedure, making it feasible to undertake multivessel percutaneous coronary revascularization with acceptable peri-procedural risks. Clinical trials are under way to compare intra-coronary stenting with bypass surgery in patients with multivessel coronary artery disease.[4] Other studies are assessing the impact of re-opening an occluded infarct-related artery on left ventricular remodelling in asymptomatic post-MI patients.[5] The results of these studies will identify the subsets of post-MI patients who are likely to gain most benefit from invasive investigation.

Dyspnoea

Impaired left ventricular systolic function post-MI predisposes to clinical cardiac failure and the one-year mortality of patients with new onset cardiac failure in the community is in excess of 25%. In a patient with exertional dyspnoea, transthoracic echocardiography should be used to confirm left ventricular systolic dysfunction. This is important because up to 50% of patients on heart failure treatment may have no evidence of cardiac dysfunction.[6] Furthermore, in those with left ventricular dysfunction (LVD), less than one-half receive appropriate therapy.

There is clear evidence to support the use of angiotensin converting enzyme (ACE) inhibitors among patients with left ventricular systolic dysfunction, to delay the appearance of symptoms, prevent worsening of symptoms and reduce the risk of recurrent hospital admission.[7–9] More importantly, ACE inhibitors have been shown to reduce mortality in post-infarct patients with heart failure by up to 40%; they are also associated with a trend towards a reduction in MI.[6]

Emerging data support the use of angiotensin-II receptor antagonists for improving symptoms and reducing the rate of worsening cardiac failure;[10] further studies are also under way to define their role more clearly, particularly their effect on mortality. β-blockers also reduce morbidity and mortality in selected patients with mild to moderate heart failure. Trials under way will define both the optimum doses and the patient subgroups who are likely to gain benefit from pharmacological therapy for heart failure.[11]

Surgery has a limited, but potentially expanding, role in the treatment of heart failure. When exertional dyspnoea is an anginal equivalent, patients with reversible ischaemia (associated with multivessel coronary artery disease and impaired left ventricular function) can benefit from coronary revascularization. In severe heart failure, donor organ shortage restricts the availability of cardiac transplant to a very small minority of patients; genetically engineered pig hearts may, however, change this in the future. Finally, the concept of myocardial viability — with the recognition that LVD due to 'stunned' or 'hibernating' myocardium can be reversible — has led to rapid advances in developing markers to detect viable myocardium and to identify patients who might benefit from surgical revascularization.[12]

Palpitation

Coronary artery disease accounts for over 80% of all sudden unexplained deaths. About 50% of these are not associated with acute plaque rupture, but occur in the presence of scarring from previous MI. Ventricular arrhythmias are strongly implicated in the aetiology of sudden death. Post-MI patients presenting with palpitation should therefore be investigated with 24-hour ambulatory electrocardiography, or patient-activated devices such as the cardiomemo or implanted 'reveal' loop recorders. Referral to an electrophysiologist for programmed electrical ventricular stimulation should be considered to identify patients who might benefit from appropriately tailored therapy.

Ventricular tachycardia and fibrillation can either be suppressed by anti-arrhythmic therapy or terminated by the implantable cardioverter defibrillator. In a recent meta-analysis of 13 trials, involving 6,500 patients with recent MI or congestive heart failure, prophylactic amiodarone was associated with a 13% (95% CI 1–22) reduction in total mortality and a 29% (95% CI 15–41) reduction in arrhythmic or sudden death.[13] The risk of arrhythmic death was highest in patients with symptomatic cardiac failure; it is therefore likely that the greatest absolute benefit of amiodarone will occur among such patients.

Recent trials comparing the cardioverter defibrillator with anti-arrhythmic therapy have also shown impressive reductions in mortality, with the defibrillator, of up to 54%.[14] A criticism of these small trials is that they represent a minority of highly selected patients, for example, patients with ejection faction <40%, in whom ventricular arrhythmias could be induced at electrophysiological testing despite drug therapy. The defibrillator trials did not have a placebo group and therefore a pro-arrhythmic effect of the drug cannot be excluded; also patients receiving β-blockers in the defibrillator arm may obscure the true benefit of the device.[15] Further studies in a broader spectrum of patients will assess the usefulness of the cardioverter defibrillator in post-infarct patients with premature ventricular contractions or couplets and in patients with class II or III heart failure.[15]

Pre-infarction patients

The impact of hospital interventions on mortality is limited because the majority of deaths from acute MI occur in the community before the patient reaches hospital. Improvement in out-of-hospital resuscitation and a reduction in delay in calling for help deserve attention but, as yet, these measures have had limited impact on reducing overall mortality from MI.

Going further back in the natural history of the disease, the identification of patients in the weeks or months leading up to to the acute event could potentially have a large impact on reducing overall infarct mortality. The occurrence of prodromal angina two or more months before MI has been known about for

Figure 2: Scheme for early investigation of new patients with suspected angina

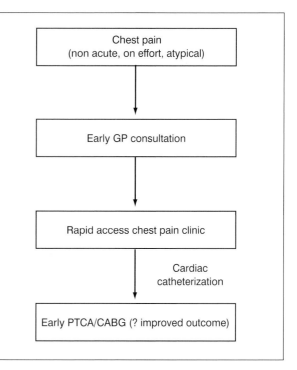

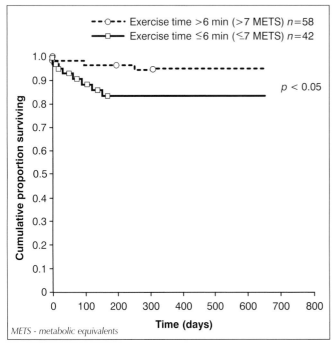

METS - metabolic equivalents

Figure 3:
Risk stratification of new patients presenting with typical angina in general practice according to exercise duration[20]

over 60 years. Prospective data from a unique chest pain clinic, specifically dedicated to investigating the outcome of new onset angina in the community, suggest that 11% of patients presenting to their GP with angina are likely to experience MI or death within one year of presentation; a further 22% undergo coronary revascularization.[16] The Southampton study was the first to demonstrate prospectively the feasibility of using a rapid access chest pain clinic to identify high-risk new angina patients representative of those presenting in general practice.[16] This approach has been supported by numerous retrospective audits of other chest pain clinics in the UK.[17–19]

Public education can increase awareness about cardiac chest pain among high-risk groups, such as middle-aged men and women with cardiovascular risk factors. Through this, patients with non-acute chest pain are encouraged to seek advice from their GP at an earlier stage in the natural history of their disease. Immediate referral by the GP to a rapid access chest pain clinic enables assessment of the patient within 48 hours by a cardiologist (Figure 2). A simple treadmill exercise test can identify new patients with angina who may benefit from early cardiac catheterization and, where appropriate, coronary revascularization.[20] Figure 3 shows that an exercise duration of $\leq$ 6 minutes on the Bruce protocol treadmill test was independently associated with reduced event-free survival from fatal and non-fatal MI during the first year after presentation.[20] Whether revascularization early in the natural history of symptomatic coronary artery disease reduces mortality from MI requires evaluation through a randomized controlled trial.

Conclusion

Any patient in the community who develops cardiovascular symptoms following MI, should be investigated regardless of age. This will enable clarification of diagnosis and also facilitate selection for effective therapeutic interventions to reduce morbidity and mortality. An additional key group to target are patients presenting for the first time to their GP with suspected angina, usually indicating an increased risk of MI. Earlier referral of such patients to a rapid access chest pain clinic for assessment by a cardiologist could reduce mortality and the frequency of adverse outcomes associated with MI.

References

1. Gandhi MM. Clinical epidemiology of coronary heart disease in the UK. *Br J Hosp Med* 1997; **58**: 23–7.

2. Kurbaan A, Bowker T, Rickards A. Pills, balloons or the knife: a review of the trials. *Heart* 1997; **78**(suppl 2): 2–5.

3. Gandhi MM, Dawkins KD. Intracoronary stents. *BMJ* 1999; **318**: 650–3.

4. Serruys P, Unger F, Van Herwerden L *et al*. Arterial Revascularisation Therapy Study: The ARTS study, a randomised trial of bypass surgery versus stenting in multivessel coronary disease. *Circulation* 1998; **98**(suppl 1): 1–498.

5. Yousef Z, Bucknall C, Webb-Peploe M, Marber M. Late opening of the infarct related artery - effect on exercise tolerance and quality of life: preliminary results of the open artery trial (TOAT study). *Circulation* 1998; **98**(suppl 1): 2273.

6. Cleland J, Swedberg K, Poole-Wilson P. Successes and failures of the current treatment of heart failure. *Lancet* 1998; **352**: 19–28.

7. Yusuf S, Nicklas J, Timmis G *et al*. Effect of enalapril on mortality and the development of heart failure in asymptomatic patients with reduced left ventricular ejection fractions. *N Engl J Med* 1992; **327**: 685–91.

8. Pfeffer M, Braunwald E, Moye L *et al*. Effect of captopril on mortality and morbidity in patients with left ventricular dysfunction after myocardial infarction - results of the survival and ventricular enlargement trials. *N Engl J Med* 1992; **327**: 669–77.

9. Yusuf S. Effect of enalapril on survival in patients with reduced left ventricular ejection fractions and congestive heart failure. *N Engl J Med* 1991; **325**: 293–302.

10. Crozier I, Ikram H, Awan M *et al*. Losartan in heart failure: haemodynamic effects and tolerability. *Circulation* 1995; **91**: 691–97.

11. Krumholz H. β-blockers for mild to moderate heart failure. *Lancet* 1999; **353**: 2.

12. Marwick TH. The viable myocardium: epidemiology, detection and clinical implications. *Lancet* 1998; **351**: 815–9.

13. Amiodarone Trials Meta-analysis Investigators. Effect of prophylactic amiodarone on mortality after acute myocardial infarction and in congestive heart failure: meta-analysis of individual data from 6,500 patients in randomised trials. *Lancet* 1997; **350**: 417–24.

14. Moss AJ, Hall WJ, Cannom DS *et al*. Improved survival with an implanted defibrillator in patients with coronary disease at high risk from ventricular arrhythmia. *N Engl J Med* 1996; **335**: 1933–40.

15. Myerburg R, Castellanos A. Clinical trials of implantable defibrillators. *N Engl J Med* 1997; **337**: 1621–3.

16. Gandhi MM, Lampe FC, Wood DA. Incidence, clinical characteristics, and short term prognosis of angina pectoris. *Br Heart J* 1995; **73**: 193–8.

17. Jain D, Fluck D, Sayer J *et al*. One-stop chest pain clinic can identify high cardiac risk. *J R Coll Physicians Lond* 1997; **31**: 401–4.

18. Newby D, Fox K, Flint L, Boon N. 'Same day' direct-access chest pain clinic: improved management and reduced hospitalisation. *Q J Med* 1998; **91**: 333–7.

19. Davie A, Caesar D, Caruana L *et al*. Outcome from a rapid-assessment chest pain clinic. *Q J Med* 1998; **91**: 339–43.

20. Gandhi MM. *Angina pectoris and ambulatory myocardial ischaemia in the general population.* Glasgow: University of Glasgow MD Thesis, 1994.

Cardiac rehabilitation and secondary prevention

Jane Flint, Dudley Group of Hospitals NHS Trust, West Midlands

The aim of the rehabilitation community — to provide a seamless service from the acute hospital setting into long-term community follow-up — is today given more impetus than ever before by the need to ensure an effective secondary prevention network. The increasing focus within rehabilitation on this key clinical goal of secondary prevention should not, however, detract from the wider aim of improved quality of life which, although difficult to measure, also contributes to the secondary prevention target. The major components of this are smoking cessation, exercise prescription, lipid and weight monitoring, blood pressure control and stress management.

Beginning with the Joint British Recommendations,[1] published this year, this paper will examine the following: a prevention and rehabilitation programme model, a recent literature survey, the current issues in the UK (with evidence from the British Association for Cardiac Rehabilitation (BACR) UK database[2]) and, finally, the primary and secondary care interface within the community. De Bono recently introduced an editorial with these words:

'Ten minutes of structured consultant time in the context of a rehabilitation process may be more valuable and more cost effective than an isolated 10 minutes in the middle of a busy outpatient clinic'.[3]

There is a clear need for cardiologists — particularly those with district responsibility — to become the team leaders of their developing multidisciplinary services for both rehabilitation and secondary prevention.

Joint British Recommendations

The Joint British Recommendations on the prevention of coronary heart disease (CHD) in clinical practice recommend that, in the hospital sector, the care of coronary and other vascular disease patients should embrace all aspects of secondary prevention and cardiac rehabilitation. This integrated service should then be available to all patients across the interface between primary and secondary care, to ensure optimal long-term management.

Blood pressure and cholesterol

The British Hypertension Society has now lowered the target blood pressure for secondary prevention in CHD in the wake of the recently published hypertension optimal treatment (HOT) study to <140/85 mmHg.[1,4] The British Hyperlipidaemia Association has re-emphasized the need for a target total cholesterol of <5.0 mmol/l.[1] Further practical clarification of management for a patient presenting with an acute coronary syndrome advises that, for an inpatient, if total cholesterol is ≥6.0 mmol/l then statin therapy should be started immediately; in addition they should be placed on a low fat diet.[1] If total cholesterol is between 5.0–6.0 mmol/l then a low fat diet should be instituted and a lipid profile repeated at six weeks; if cholesterol remains >5.0 mmol/l after three months of a low fat diet, then statin therapy should be initiated. Finally, cholesterol levels should be checked annually in patients with CHD if the starting level is <5.0 mmol/l.[1]

Diabetes mellitus

Earlier and stricter control of diabetes mellitus has been re-emphasized this year. Diabetic patients, even in the absence of established CHD, should have their risk factors managed in

33

the same way as in a non-diabetic patient with a past history of myocardial infarction (MI). Angiotensin-converting enzyme inhibitors, statins or β-blockers may all be of particular benefit in the treatment of ischaemic heart disease in patients with diabetes mellitus. The target blood pressure for diabetic patients should be <130/80 mm/Hg.[1,4]

Prevention and rehabilitation programme model

An ideal prevention and rehabilitation programme model includes four phases, with a protocol in place for longer-term surveillance. It should emphasize the integration of all stages, together with longer-term surveillance needs, as the rate of progression of coronary heart disease is so variable. Phase I refers to the inpatient phase of acute MI or other coronary syndrome. In the UK we tend to perform some pre-discharge risk assessment and individual counselling regarding risk factors, diet, exercise and vocational commitments.

Phase II refers to the early outpatient phase, but may also include some of the phase I services. More support is now being given than has traditionally been the case; this ideally involves a cardiac liaison nurse working in the community following Post Coronary Care Unit (PCCU) discharge. In addition to practical monitoring, these nurses are also well-versed in the psychosocial aspects of care. Phase III classes include exercise prescription as well as other counselling by various multidisciplinary professionals, with clinical input where required. Phase IV refers to maintenance of exercise habit and, hopefully, other lifestyle changes and control of risk factors; this phase clearly needs to be linked into medical care in the community and across the primary/secondary care interface.

Surveillance of CHD patients is an area where more guidelines are required in view of the variable course of the disease. Our own Dudley rehabilitation and prevention network includes the Action Heart programme. Research by Dugmore *et al* has revealed significant changes in cardiorespiratory fitness, psychological well-being, quality of life and vocational status, following a one-year cardiac exercise rehabilitation programme.[5] This involves an exercise test at enrolment and again after six months and one year on the programme.

The length of the standard programme has recently been reduced from 24 to 12 months, having established by audit that maintenance of exercise habit is likely to be achieved by this stage.[6] Our Phase IV health club, closely allied to Action Heart, continues for as long as the patients wish to attend. The basic Phase III programme involves circuit interval training three times a week and at least the first three sessions are monitored by telemetry, longer for higher risk individuals. Advice on diet, lifestyle and stress management is given and, over the last two years, we have also developed an adjacent seminar programme which may involve patients not wishing to undertake the exercise component.

It is important that we encourage the attendance of patients from minority groups, including ethnic minorities and the elderly, as they are likely to gain most benefit. Patients who deteriorate during the course of the two-year Action Heart programme are subject to further investigation. If coronary angiography is not immediately indicated by an early positive test, then myocardial perfusion imaging is used to define the exact extent of the myocardium at ischaemic risk; the need for angiography and intervention can then be assessed.[7]

Literature focus

The overviews of cardiac rehabilitation,[8] which established mortality benefits in the late 1980s and the 1992 British Cardiac Society (BCS) working party report[9] recommending its widespread uptake, gave birth to the publication of guidelines by BACR and others.[10] In recent years the literature has focused on two aspects of practice — psychosocial and risk factor management.

Psychosocial aspects

A patient's initial perception of their illness is an important determinant of their post-MI recovery.[11] Deprived patients are invited, but are significantly less likely to attend, rehabilitation.[12] Data from our own group confirmed a lower rate from poorer social groups, but compliance for attenders was, encouragingly, very evenly distributed.[13] Two negative studies of early psychosocial intervention in recent years have raised criticism, but an overview by Linden et al,[14] which showed that good psychosocial counselling could aid stress reduction and quality of life improvement. Mayou[15] then stated that there should be psychologically-informed early routine care for all patients, plus additional care for selected patients; it should be flexible and also integrated with primary care and cardiac aftercare.

Risk factor management

De Busk et al[16] found that a dedicated home-based case management system, led by medically directed nurses, was considerably more effective than the usual medical care as in and out patients for modification of risk factors post-MI. We know how sub-optimal recording and management of risk factors can be from the action on secondary prevention through intervention to reduce events (ASPIRE) survey.[17] The Euro ASPIRE data also confirmed the under-use of secondary preventative drug treatment. In early 1998 Lewin et al [18] criticized limited assessments made; however the BACR UK database does show significant ability to document and audit and this should be positively encouraged. We know that cardiac rehabilitation post-MI can be as cost-effective in quality of life terms as coronary bypass surgery (CABG) for severe angina and left main stem disease, as Oldridge's recent review indicates.[19] The August Effective Health Care Bulletin on cardiac rehabilitation[20] is unfortunately anachronistic in neglecting important networking with secondary prevention.

Current issues in the UK

A recent Royal College of Physicians survey[21] has shown that, in phase I, 70% of acute cases of MI are still formally managed under general physicians. This is clearly an area that needs attention, as this phase often determines the standard or absence of cardiac aftercare and rehabilitation. There is a need for individually planned secondary prevention, based on good risk and rehabilitation assessment and with recognition of psychosocial needs. Patients transferred to tertiary centres may require more consideration, but often in fact receive less, due to the intervention demands of the centre.

Phase II may become the waiting list for phase III, but can be enriched by visits by general practitioners (GPs) or community cardiac liaison nurses, seminar programmes and helplines. It is likely that the Heart manual may find a niche here with a good facilitator.[22] Phase III typically lasts between six-12 weeks but can be extended if necessary. A Scottish study by Campbell et al[23] found that less than 20% of suitable patients attend rehabilitation, reflecting a poor phase I-II referral rate. Clearly support is needed beyond phase III; at present most phase IV experience is an extension of phase III programmes that last for more then a year. There is a need for programmes that will keep patients on, as rising referral rates increase the demand for phase IV within the community.

The BACR now runs a phase IV training module, for exercise professionals with sufficient exercise teaching background; in addition, qualified health professionals are also being encouraged to undertake training. Referral protocols are in place for phase III-IV handovers, to ensure that adequate risk assessment has taken place and that there are secondary prevention plans for individual patients. The BACR has a vision of health and exercise professionals joining forces with medical backup to promote quality phase IV community programmes, such as those that exist in Europe and the US. It is also essential that financial issues do not compromise standards of surveillance. Good communication is the key to a good programme; the use of a shared care card, pioneered in Glasgow for control of hypertension, may also be helpful. Finally, a system of follow-up that is flexible and appropriate for individual needs should also be established.

British Association for Cardiac Rehabilitation UK database

The BACR UK Database[2] now has recorded entries of 300 cardiac rehabilitation programmes — more than any other UK survey. Most are hospital-based (68%), 19% are both hospital- and community-based and just 9% are solely community-based. Programmes are coordinated by nurses in 79%, physiotherapists in 14%, occupational therapists in 4% and doctors in just 3%. The results of risk-assessment programmes are as follows: out of 246 responders, 175 (71%) were risk-assessed both pre and post-rehabilitation, 50 (20%) were only pre-assessed, 3 (1%) were only post-assessed and 18 (7%) were not assessed at all. With regard to exercise assessment, 40% undertook some form before their rehabilitation programme but only 22% both before and after the programme, 7% only afterwards.

It appears that the facility to record data is present in most courses, despite Lewin's recent figures.[18] Of the 300 centres assessed, 235 reported some form of ongoing audit; however, a need was highlighted for greater emphasis on risk factor management. Most centres were found to employ a multidisciplinary team: 95% use nurses, 82% physiotherapists, 50% dietitians and 43% doctors; a lesser percentage also use pharmacists (31%), occupational therapists (28%), exercise physiologists (14%) and psychologists (12%). In a few (less than 5%) cases vocational counsellors and social workers are also available. Of all the phase III programmes, 59% offer, or say they provide, a link to phase IV programmes, clearly establishing the close relationship that these two phases should have. The Heart manual is used in 22% of programmes, although its place is still currently being evaluated and defined through ongoing research.[22] It is currently employed mainly in remote areas some distance from the local hospital, or in other regions where it has been promoted. Soon it may well find a general place for use in straightforward cases.

Secondary prevention/rehabilitation network

A telephone survey[24] of the BACR UK database between April and July 1998 questioned each centre about their secondary prevention networks. These include PCCUs and various modes of follow-up, including dedicated post-MI, cardiologist and secondary prevention clinics. Knowledge of local heart disease strategy for secondary prevention, secondary prevention protocols and community nurse and other efforts were tested.

Of the 300 units contacted — comprising district and regional clinical rehabilitation centres and community rehabilitation/clinic programmes — 240 (80%) responded to the questionnaire. Most programmes (70%) were aware that secondary prevention was included in the district heart disease strategy (negotiated between the Public Health Department and clinical cardiology service) and one-half considered there to be some protocol with GPs in their district. Just under one-half (108 or 46%) knew of a lipid clinic in their area with considerable, but not exclusive, overlap with cardiological services and 99 (41%) were associated with a clinical service, involving majority cardiological cover and follow-up of patients post-MI.[24]

An overall impression of network development was inferred from all data, as was the ability to describe a pathway of cardiac care with good risk assessment and integrated management between hospital and community. Of the programmes contacted, 88 (38%) provided a coronary rehabilitation/secondary preventive network, but 77 (32%) did not; 37 (15%) were developing some form of network and another 37 (15%) provide one to some extent in the community.

Compared with this, a questionnaire administered to general practices in Dudley found 28 (58%) with no specific secondary prevention facility as yet, just six (18%) having a GP or nurse secondary prevention clinic and only seven (21%) clearly stating that the hospital outpatient department was used. Only one practice (3%) was due to set up a specific facility. Among those 28 without facilities, seven had some plans, eight had possible plans and 13 had no plans.[24]

Conclusion

Results of the BACR UK database survey reflect the haphazard nature of secondary prevention practice within the community.[25] Both rehabilitation and secondary prevention feature prominently in government documents, including the emerging National Service Framework, and this will hopefully ensure the securement of resources. Given the current economic constraints, cardiologists, as team leaders, must make their case forcefully. Primary care groups are just forming and the timing of the British Recommendations on Prevention[1] may be quite strategic. Nurse-prescribing by protocol is on the horizon and will undoubtedly benefit patients. The exact context of healthy living centres is just being defined and the National Health Service Executive has been involved in phase IV development discussions. Finally, it is essential that district general hospital cardiologists are experts in preventative and rehabilitation cardiology.[26]

References

1. Wood D, Durrington P, Poulter N et al on behalf of the British Cardiac Society, British Hyperlipidaemia Association, British Hypertension Society and British Diabetic Association. Joint British recommendations on prevention of coronary heart disease in clinical practice. *Heart* 1998; **80**(suppl 2).

2. Bethell H, Turner SC, Flint EJ, Rose I. The BACR UK database of cardiac rehabilitation units, secondary prevention networks in the UK prevention networks. 1999. In press.

3. De Bono D. Models of cardiac rehabilitation [Editorial]. *BMJ* 1998; **316**: 1329.

4. Hansson L, Zanchetti A, Carruthers SG et al. Effects of intensive blood presure lowering and low-dose aspirin in patients with hypertension: principal results of the hypertension optimal treatment (HOT) randomised trial. *Lancet* 1998; **351**: 1755–62.

5. Dugmore LD, Tidson RJ, Phillips MH et al. Changes in cardio-respiratory fitness, psychological well-being, quality of life and vocational status following a 12-month cardiac exercise rehabilitation programme. *Heart* 1999. In press.

6. Edmunds E, Higginson E, Flint EJ et al. Cardiac rehabilitation: are 24 months better than 12 for exercise benefit? *Proc Cardiovasc Prevention* 1998; **4**:

7. Shipsey J, Wong K, Flint J et al. Use of Thallium 201 myocardial scintigraphy in monitoring deteriorating exercise tests during a long-term rehabilitation programme. [Astract]. *Nucl Med Commun* 1994; **10**: 258–9.

8. Oldridge N, Guyatt GH, Fischer ME et al. Cardiac rehabilitation after myocardial infarction. Combined experience of randomised clinical trials. *JAMA* 1988; **260**: 945–50.

9. Horgan, Bethell H, Carson P et al. Working party report on cardiac rehabilitation. *Brit Heart J* 1992; **67**: 412–18.

10. Thompson D, Bowmans GS, De Bono DP et al. *Cardiac rehabilitation: guidelines and audit standards.* London: Royal College of Physicians, 1997.

11. Petrie KJ, Weinman J, Sharpe N et al. Role of patients view of their illness in predicting return to work and functioning after myocardial infarction: longitudinal study. *BMJ* 1996; **312**: 1191–4.

12. Pell J, Pell A, Morrison C et al. Retrospective study of influence of deprivation on up-take of cardiac rehabilitation. *BMJ* 1996; **313**: 267–8.

13. Tipson R, Welsh AL, Evans RE et al. Are referral and drop out rates to cardiac rehabilitation programmes subject to health inequalities? A 25 month audit of the Action Heart cardiac rehabilitation programme. *Proc Brit Assoc Cardiac Rehab* 1998; **1**(4): 1369–3972.

14. Linden W, Stossel C, Maurice J et al. Psychosocial interventions for patients with coronary artery disease: a meta-analysis. *Arch Intern Med* 1996; **156**: 1745–52.

15. Mayou R. Rehabilitation after heart attack. *BMJ* 1996; **313**: 1498–9.

16. DeBusk R, Miller NH, Superko R et al. A case management system for coronary risk factor modification after acute myocardial infarction. *Ann Intern Med* 1994; **120**: 721–9.

17. ASPIRE steering group. British Cardiac Society survey of the potential for secondary prevention of coronary heart disease. *Heart* 1996; **75**: 334–42.

18. Lewin RJP, Ingleton R, Newens AJ et al. Adherence to cardiac rehabilitation guidelines: a survey of cardiac rehabilitation programmes in the UK. *BMJ* 1998; **316**: 1354–5.

19. Oldridge N. Cardiac rehabilitation and risk factor management after myocardial infarction: clinical and economic evaluation. *Wien Klin Wochenschr* 1997; **109**: 6–16.

20. *Cardiac rehabilitation.* Effective Health Care Bulletin 4, Number 4. York: NHS Centre for Reviews and Dissemination, 1998.

21. Mather. *Impact of change in training on acute medical services. Royal College of Physicians Survey.* London: Royal College of Physicians, 1998.

22. Bell J. *Personal communication,*1998. Thesis.

23. Campbell NC, Grimshaw JM, Ritchie LD *et al.* Outpatient cardiac rehabilitation: are the potential benefits being realised? *J Roy Coll Phys* 1996; **30**: 14–9.

24. Flint EJ, Lamb P, Higginson EJ. *Secondary prevention/cardiac rehabilitation networks across the primary secondary care interface. Proc Brit Assoc Cardiac Rehab* 1998; **1**: 4.

25. Campbell NC, Thains J, Deans HG *et al.* Secondary prevention clinics for coronary heart disease: randomised trial of effect on health. *BMJ* 1998; **316**: 1434–7.

26. Working party for British Cardiac Society on interface between District General Hospital and regional centre. *Heart* 1997; **78**: 522.

Secondary prevention: pharmacology

Michael Schachter, Imperial College School of Medicine, St Mary's Hospital, London

Over the past few years much has been learnt about the means of improving both survival rates and quality of life for patients following myocardial infarction (MI) but, for a variety of reasons, the lessons have been less widely applied than was initially intended.

This paper will assess some of the available evidence for pharmacological approaches to secondary prevention and will focus, in particular, on several recent reviews.[1–3] It is important to bear in mind that pharmacological treatment is only a part of the process, which should also include changes in lifestyle and other non-pharmacological approaches — issues addressed elsewhere in this book.

Rationale for drug therapies in secondary prevention

The treatments most commonly used following acute MI can be broadly classed under the following headings:

- anti-arrhythmic agents
- anti-platelet and anticoagulant drugs
- lipid-lowering drugs
- drugs which preserve or improve left ventricular function (LVF).

There are also various other treatments used and these will be considered after the four main categories.

Anti-arrhythmic agents

β-blockers have been the outstanding success in this area and, some might suggest, the only one.[4] Of course, their action extends beyond anti-arrhythmic properties, since they also reduce cardiac work by lowering contractility, heart rate and sometimes also blood pressure. Acute treatment with β-blockers, starting within 24 hours post-MI using intravenous therapy and continuing for a week, reduces short-term mortality by about 13–15%. Several large chronic studies, lasting from three months to three years, have suggested improvements in survival of 20–40%, with a particularly striking effect in reducing sudden deaths.[5] This provides at least circumstantial evidence for an anti-arrhythmic effect.

The cardioselectivity of the β-blocker does not appear to be relevant in determining efficacy. It is an apparent paradox, given orthodox teaching about these drugs, that it is patients with large infarcts and impaired LVF who benefit most from β-blockade. However, uncompensated heart failure remains a contraindication, as does bradyarrhythmia and hypotension. Treatment should be continued for at least two to three years if well tolerated and possibly indefinitely. It should be noted that β-blockers retain their usefulness in diabetic patients, despite the reservations usually associated with them in this group. The authors of a recent retrospective survey of over 200,000 MI survivors suggested that there should be virtually no exclusions,[6] but the evidence for this was inconclusive compared to a randomized controlled trial.[7]

By contrast, the type I anti-arrhythmic drugs have proved very disappointing. The Cardiac Arrhythmias Suppression Trial (CAST) in post-infarct patients with ventricular ectopics suggested that flecainide and encainide actually increased mortality, presumably (but not definitely) because of pro-arrhythmic effects.[8] Two trials with amiodarone in Europe and Canada have been more promising, but criteria for identification of suitable patients remain unclear. Given the many side-effects, this is not a drug that should be used on a routine basis until patient selection is better understood.

Anti-platelet and anticoagulant drugs

Aspirin has become the drug most closely associated with post-MI secondary prevention. Some 40 trials have now established its efficacy in patients with proven cardiovascular disease, although not all of these were MI survivors. There is a reduction of about 25% in cardiovascular events and a somewhat smaller reduction in mortality. The largest effect is in reducing stroke incidence. [9,10] Although early trials used doses of over 1 g per day, the dose more recently recommended is 75–300 mg daily. This appears to be equally effective with fewer side-effects although, even at the lower dose, there is an increased risk of gastrointestinal and other bleeding. It is possible that even lower doses may be effective but this is, as yet, unproven. The CAPRIE trial has shown that the new anti-platelet drug clopidogrel is comparable in efficacy and safety to aspirin, but is of course far more expensive.[11] Its role in secondary prevention may be largely confined to patients who are intolerant of aspirin, but it is too early to draw definite conclusions.

The use of warfarin and related anticoagulants in secondary prevention remains a controversial issue. Several trials have shown worthwhile reductions in reinfarction and stroke (between 30% and 55%), though with less marked effects on mortality and with a significant risk of intracranial haemorrhage.[12] There is currently no evidence that warfarin is superior to aspirin although, surprisingly, true direct comparison is still lacking in this group of patients. Warfarin is therefore not routinely used in post-infarct patients, though some clinicians use it frequently, especially in patients with atrial fibrillation or mural thrombus.

Lipid-lowering drugs

Perhaps it is in the area of lipid-lowering therapy that the most dramatic change in clinical thinking has taken place in the last five years. The crucial event was the publication of the Scandinavian Simvastatin Survival Study (4S) of over 4,000 patients who had angina or previous MI.[13] This showed a reduction of 30% in total mortality over five years, mostly attributable to a 42% reduction in coronary deaths. The incidence of coronary events fell by 34% and there was a similar decrease in revascularization procedures. In this population the range of plasma cholesterol was above average, between 5.5 and 8.0 mmol/l, and there were reductions of nearly 30% in total cholesterol and nearly 40% in low-density lipoprotein (LDL) cholesterol. Very importantly, there was no excess of non-cardiovascular deaths, previously the subject of not entirely rational controversy.

In the CARE (Cholesterol and Recurrent Events)[14] trial, involving over 4,000 MI survivors and using pravastatin (another HMG CoA reductase inhibitor), the mean cholesterol of 5.4 mmol/l was typical for Western societies, with an upper limit set at only 6.2 mmol/l. The reduction in total mortality over five years was more modest, at 9%, but there was still a 24% reduction in coronary deaths and non-fatal MI, with a fall of 27% in revascularization. There appeared to be a threshold at an LDL cholesterol of 3.2 mmol/l, below which statin treatment did not produce benefit; however numbers in this category were relatively small. An even larger Australasian study (LIPID) of over 9,000 patients with average cholesterol levels, all post-MI or with angina, has produced very similar results.[15]

Although the fibrates have actually been in clinical use for longer than the statins, there is as yet no comparable secondary prevention trial. However, one large-scale trial, the Bezafibrate Infarction Prevention (BIP) study, which included 3,122 post-MI and angina patients, showed bezafibrate 400 mg to have no significant effect on fatal or non-fatal MI cases or sudden death. A smaller trial, the Bezafibrate Atherosclerosis Intervention Trial (BECAIT),[16] which involved only about 90 patients with primarily angiographic endpoints, suggested a reduced incidence of coronary events (there were no deaths). As expected, there was a greater effect on triglycerides than on cholesterol (reduced by 31% against 9%). This may be important in view of the increasing recognition that triglycerides are an important cardiovascular risk factor.

Treatment which preserves or improves LVF

Angiotensin converting enzyme (ACE) inhibitors have so far proved the most successful class of drugs from this perspective. Post-MI heart size, specifically left ventricular volume, often increases and this is associated with deteriorating myocardial function and poor prognosis. Experimental evidence has indicated that this harmful remodelling could be inhibited by ACE inhibitors, which has led to great interest in their therapeutic potential.[17]

The trials now completed include both those in which post-MI patients were selected because they were at increased risk (overt heart failure, ejection fraction <40%, anterior infarction, decreased wall movement) and others in which post-MI patients were included without selection.[18,19] Perhaps not surprisingly, benefit was much greater in high-risk patients, with reductions in mortality of 20–30%, compared to less than 10% in unselected patients. Interestingly, the trials in high-risk patients also suggested that the reinfarction rate was reduced, prompting consideration of the possible anti-atherogenic activity of ACE inhibitors.[20] The benefit of treatment is maintained for three to five years, with no indication of a cut-off point at which treatment should be discontinued.

Overall, the case for using these drugs in at least the high-risk MI survivors is very strong. Their use is also arguable for all patients without specific contraindications (history of angioedema with an ACE inhibitor, bilateral renal artery stenosis and hypotension). The benefits appear to be in addition to that seen with β-blockers,[21] although this probably does not apply to all patients.[22] Presumably similar trials using angiotensin II receptor antagonists will report within a few years.

Other cardiovascular drugs

Calcium channel blockers would appear to have considerable promise in secondary prevention. Some have anti-arrhythmic properties, all can reduce cardiac preload and afterload and they too may have anti-atherogenic properties. In fact, trial results have been distinctly discouraging. Nifedipine treatment showed no benefit and one case even revealed a trend towards a less favourable outcome.[23,24] It is worth noting that these studies used short-acting formulations and there are, as yet, no comparable data on longer-acting vasoselective dihydropyridines, such as amlodipine and felodipine.

Results with the non-dihydropyridines have been less negative, possibly because they tend to slow the heart rather than causing sympathetic activation.[25] One study with diltiazem suggested a reduction in mortality and cardiac events only in patients with ejection fractions >40%, without X-ray evidence of pulmonary congestion and possibly those with non-Q wave infarcts.[26] In patients with pulmonary oedema, mortality actually increased. Two trials using verapamil have confirmed that event rates can be reduced in patients with relatively well-preserved LVF.[27,28] However, routine use of verapamil or diltiazem has not been widely accepted in secondary prevention, though one potential role may be in patients where β-blockers are contraindicated — asthma for example.

It has been shown that nitrates have no definite benefits post-MI, but they can be safely given to patients with persisting ischaemia.[29] An enhancement of the protective action of ACE inhibition has been suggested in one trial, but the evidence is unconvincing.[30]

New approaches

There is evidence that hormone replacement therapy, specifically with oestrogens, may be an effective mode of primary prevention in post-menopausal women. The Heart and Estrogen/Progestogen Replacement Study (HERS)[31] involved over 2,700 post-menopausal women with coronary artery disease, although only 17% had proven MI. Patients were given combination therapy with conjugated equine oestrogens and medroxyprogesterone, or placebo, with a mean follow-up of about four years. It was concluded that there was no beneficial effect on cardiac death rates, non-fatal MI or other cardiovascular events, but that there was an increase in venous thromboembolism and gall bladder disease. There was, however, a trend towards cardiovascular benefit over time. Trials of longer duration are required to determine the role of hormone replacement therapy in the longer term.

The concept that antioxidants may contribute to the primary and secondary prevention of cardiovascular disease has obvious appeal. This is particularly so if the antioxidants are readily available in the diet. The Cambridge Heart Antioxidant Study (CHAOS)[32] showed a reduction in non-fatal MI rates in patients with ischaemic heart disease on high-dose vitamin E (800 IU/day). There was, however, no improvement in cardiovascular mortality. Other studies are in progress to attempt to clarify this issue.

Research and reality

It is clear that, in the UK, the rest of Europe and elsewhere, secondary prevention is far from optimal.[33,34] There are many possible reasons for this:

- lack of adequate information on available therapies, including under-dosing
- lack of active intervention while patients are in hospital
- lack of follow-up, particularly in patients with 'full' recovery
- anxiety about prescribing costs.

This last is particularly unfortunate, because it takes a very short-term view. Prevention of heart failure, reinfarction and sudden death is, even in crudely financial terms, cost-effective. It is also important to consider that physicians will increasingly be held to account, not least by their patients, for not adhering to 'best practice'.

Conclusion

The recommendations set out in Table 1 for drug use in secondary prevention summarize current consensus (though probably not unanimity). There will, of course, be contra-indications, but the table can be applied to most situations. It also assumes that treatment will continue indefinitely. At the same time, concurrent disease — notably diabetes and hyper-tension — should be monitored and treated intensively, although there is little current evidence that this will improve outcome directly.

Table 1 is a formidable list of medication for the clinician to prescribe and, more impor-tantly, for the patient to take every day. It is possible that the list may even be expanded — with, for instance, the addition of vitamin supplements to reduce homocysteine levels. Patients should also receive extensive advice about diet, exercise and, of course, smoking, where applicable. Clearly, secondary prevention is not just an exercise in correct prescribing, but also a collaboration between patients and the health professionals who care for them.

Table 1 Current treatment recommendations

- All patients should be offered low- to moderate-dose aspirin (75–300 mg daily)
- β-blockers should be given to all patients without contraindications, preferably starting within 24 hours of the infarction
- ACE inhibitors should be given to all patients with overt or sub-clinical LVD and could arguably be given to all patients
- Lipid-lowering drugs (specifically statins) are appropriate for almost all patients, unless LDL cholesterol is less than 3.2 mmol/l
- Warfarin is not currently a routine recommendation but may be appropriate in some patients (see above)
- Non-dihydropyridine calcium channel blockers (particularly verapamil) are not considered routine therapy, but can be considered as an alternative to β-blockers in some cases

References

1. Rapaport E. Pharmacologic therapies after myocardial infarction. *Am J Med* 1996; **101**(suppl 4A): 61–70S.

2. Mehta RH, Eagle KA. Secondary prevention in myocardial infarction. *BMJ* 1998; **316**: 838–42.

3. Kendall MJ, Horton RC, eds. *Preventing coronary disease, cardioprotective therapeutics in practice.* 2nd ed. London: Martin Dunitz, 1998.

4. Yusuf S, Wittes J, Freidman L. Overview of results of randomised clinical trials in heart disease: treatment following myocardial infarction. *JAMA* 1988; **260**: 2088–93.

5. Kendall MJ, Lynch KP, Hjalmarson A, Kjekhus J. β-blockers and sudden cardiac death. *Ann Intern Med* 1995; **123**: 358–67.

6. Gottlieb SS, McCarter RJ, Vogel RA. Effect of β-blockade on mortality among high-risk and low-risk patients after myocardial infarction. *N Engl J Med* 1998; **339**: 489–97.

7. Radford MJ, Krumholz HM. β-blockers after myocardial infarction—for few patients, or many? *N Engl J Med* 1998; **339**: 551–3.

8. Gheorghiade M, Goldstein S. Arrhythmia suppression in post myocardial infarction patients with special notation to the Cardiac Arrhythmia Suppression Trial (CAST). *Prog Cardiovasc Dis* 1991; **33**: 213–18.

9. Antiplatelet Trialist Collaboration. Collaborative overview of randomised trial of antiplatelet therapy, I. Prevention of death, myocardial infarction and stroke by prolonged antiplatelet therapy in various categories of patients. *BMJ* 1994; **308**: 81–106.

10. Hennekens CH. Aspirin in the treatment and prevention of cardiovascular disease. *Ann Rev Public Health* 1997; **18**: 37–49.

11. CAPRIE Steering Committee. A randomised, blind trial of clopidogrel versus aspirin in patients at risk of ischaemic events. *Lancet* 1996; **348**: 1329Ó39.

12. Effect of long-term oral anticoagulant treatment on mortality and cardiovascular morbidity after myocardial infarction. Anticoagulants in the Secondary Prevention of Events in Coronary Thrombosis (ASPECT) Research Group. *Lancet* 1994; **343**: 499–503.

13. The Scandinavian Simvastatin Survival Study Group. Randomised trial of cholesterol lowering in 4,444 patients with coronary heart disease: the Scandinavian Simvastatin Survival Study (4S). *Lancet* 1994; **344**: 1383–9.

14. Sacks FM, Pfeffer MA, Moye LA *et al.* The effect of pravastatin on coronary events after myocardial infarction in patients with average cholesterol levels. *N Engl J Med* 1996; **335**: 1001–9.

15. The Long-Term Intervention with Pravastatin in Ischaemic Disease (LIPID) Study Group. Prevention of cardio-vascular events and death with pravastatin in patients with coronary heart disease and a broad range of initial cholesterol levels. *N Engl J Med* 1998; **339**: 1349–57.

16. Ericsson C, Hamsten A, Nilsson J *et al.* Angiographic assessment of effects of bezafibrate on progression of coronary disease in young male post-infarction patients. *Lancet* 1996; **347**: 849–53.

17. Konstam MA. Role of angiotensin converting enzyme inhibitors in preventing left ventricular remodelling following myocardial infarction. *Eur Heart J* 1995; **16**(suppl K): 42–8.

18. Lonn EM, Yusuf S, Jha P *et al.* Emerging role of angiotensin converting enzyme inhibitors in cardiac and vascular protection. *Circulation* 1994; **90**: 2056–69.

19. Latini R, Maggioni AP, Flather M *et al.* ACE inhibitor use in patients with myocardial infarction: summary of evidence from clinical trials. *Circulation* 1995; **92**: 3132–7.

20. Borghi C, Ambrosioni E. Evidence-based medicine and ACE inhibition. *J Cardiovasc Pharmacol* 1998; **32**(suppl 2): S24–35.

21. Murdoch DR, McMurray JJV. ACE inhibitors in myocardial infarction. *Hospital Med* 1998; **59**: 111–15.

22. McAlister FA. Trial is needed of ACE inhibitors plus β-blockers in survivors of myocardial infarction. *BMJ* 1998; **317**: 751.

23. Wilcox RG, Hampton JR, Banks DC *et al.* Trial of early nifedipine in acute myocardial infarction. The TRENT Study. *BMJ* 1986; **293**: 1204–8.

24. Israeli SPRINT Study Group. Secondary Prevention Reinfarction Israeli Nifedipine Trial (SPRINT): a randomised intervention trial of nifedipine in patients with acute myocardial infarction. *Eur Heart J* 1988; **9**: 354–64.

25. Sleight P. Calcium antagonists during and after myocardial infarction. *Drugs* 1996; **51**: 216–25.

26. The Multicenter Diltiazem Postinfarction Trial Research Group. The effect of diltiazem on mortality and rein-farction after myocardial infarction. *N Engl J Med* 1988; **319**: 385–92.

27. Danish Study Group on Verapamil in Myocardial Infarction. The Danish studies on verapamil in myocardial infarction. *Br J Clin Pharmacol* 1986; **21**: 197–204S.

28. Danish Study Group on Verapamil in Myocardial Infarction. The effect of verapamil on mortality and major events after acute myocardial infarction. The Danish Verapamil Infarction Trial II (DAVIT-II). *Am J Cardiol* 1990; **66**: 779–85.

29. ISIS-4 (Fourth International Study of Infarct Survival) Collaborative Group. ISIS-4: a randomised factorial trial assessing early captopril, oral mononitrate, and intravenous magnesium sulphate in 58,050 patients with suspected acute myocardial infarction. *Lancet* 1995; **345**: 669–85.

30. Gruppo Italiano per lo Studio della Sopravvivenza nell'Infarcto Miocardico. Six month effects of early treatment with lisinopril and transdermal glyceryl trinitrate singly and together withdrawn six weeks after acute myocardial infarction: the GISSI-3 trial. *J Am Coll Cardiol* 1996; **27**: 337–44.

31. Hulley S, Grady D, Bush T *et al*. Randomized trial of estrogen plus progestin for secondary prevention of coronary heart disease in post-menopausal women. *JAMA* 1998; **280**: 605–13.

32. Stephens NG, Parsons A, Schofield PM *et al*. Randomised controlled trial of vitamin E in patients with coronary disease: Cambridge Heart Antioxidant Study (CHAOS). *Lancet* 1996; **347**: 781–6.

33. EUROASPIRE. A European Society of Cardiology survey of secondary prevention of coronary heart disease: principal results. *Eur Heart J* 1997; **18**: 1569–82.

34. Campbell NC, Thain J, Deans HG *et al*. Secondary prevention in coronary heart disease: baseline survey of provision in general practice. *BMJ* 1998; **316**:1430–4.

Secondary prevention: general practice

John Ferguson, Prescription Pricing Authority, Newcastle-upon-Tyne

Cardiovascular disease is multifactorial and one of the most common causes of morbidity and mortality. It is the main cause of death in the UK, accounting for some 300,000 deaths a year. There is considerable geographical variation in the death rates, which are higher in the north of England, urban areas and areas of social and economic deprivation. Differences in smoking rates and blood pressure levels do not fully explain the variation and total cholesterol levels do not vary across the country to any great extent. The present preoccupation with cholesterol testing and the availability of lipid-lowering drugs should not prevent us from taking a holistic approach to the patient. It is important to assess all the risk factors for cardiovascular disease for an individual patient and to avoid simply treating a laboratory test result.

The National Health Service (NHS) Centre for Reviews and Dissemination reminds us that cholesterol levels are a poor predictor of those who will develop heart disease. Smokers with high blood pressure are three times more likely to die from heart disease than non-smokers with low blood pressure, when both have the same cholesterol levels.[1] As a result of several high profile clinical trials[2,3] and the Department of Health's 'Health of the Nation' targets,[4] the management of the health risks associated with hyperlipidaemia have increased in importance over the past few years. This has led to an increase in the use of lipid-lowering agents.

Among the risk factors known to affect coronary heart disease (CHD) are smoking, inadequate physical activity, raised blood cholesterol levels and raised blood pressure. Risk factors are well-recognized and fall into two classes. Fixed factors include family history, sex, age and diabetes mellitus. Modifiable factors include smoking, hypertension, obesity, lack of physical exercise and high cholesterol. The intense current interest in lipids has encouraged a one-dimensional approach to coronary risk, based on pre-determined total serum cholesterol or low density lipoprotein (LDL) cholesterol cut-off points. Epidemiological evidence shows that CHD risk is multifactorial and that an individual's risk cannot be determined by considering lipid measurements in isolation.[1] The effects are not simply additive and it is the combination of factors — rather than individual factors in isolation — that need to be considered.

Treatment available

Antihypertensives

Hypertension is a major risk factor which is amenable to treatment. Thiazide diuretics and β-blockers are the only two groups of drugs for which long-term beneficial effects on morbidity and mortality have been demonstrated. Newer treatments, such as angiotensin converting enzyme (ACE) inhibitors, certainly reduce blood pressure, but their long-term effects on morbidity and mortality are not yet known. In the absence of any contraindication to thiazide diuretics or β-blockers, one of these drugs is a rational first choice. Effective treatment at all ages produces a 30% reduction in the risk of both coronary artery disease and stroke.[5]

Diuretics

The total use of diuretics remains constant. The trend has been to increase the use of thiazides and loop diuretics and there has also been a marked reduction in the use of potassium-sparing combination diuretics and diuretics combined with potassium.

Research indicates that the optimum antihypertensive effect of thiazide diuretics can be achieved with a maximum of 2.5 mgs of bendrofluazide.[6] Its use has tripled in the last five years.

β-blockers

Patients often try to avoid these drugs because they believe they cause fatigue, diminish their exercise capacity and so reduce quality of life. Research studies do not tend to support this belief and one large study recently found that the quality of life was improved with atenolol compared with placebo.[7] Over the past five years the national trend in the usage of β-blockers has remained relatively constant, atenolol and propranolol being the most frequently prescribed. There has been a small reduction in the use of the disproportionately expensive combination products with β-blockers. Over the past five years the national costs of β-blockers have fallen annually from £116m to £80m, mainly due to the reduced cost of generic atenolol. Currently there is a three-fold variation in the use of these drugs by health authorities.[8]

ACE inhibitors

ACE inhibitors, in combination with diuretics, can improve symptoms and prolong life for many heart failure patients and can also be used in the treatment of hypertension. The British Hypertension Society guidelines recommend that the use of ACE inhibitors as first-line therapy should be reserved for those patients whose medical history makes the use of conventional therapies inappropriate.[9] ACE inhibitors should be considered for hypertension when thiazides and β-blockers are contraindicated, not tolerated, or fail to control blood pressure. They are particularly indicated for the treatment of hypertension in insulin-dependent diabetics, but best avoided in patients with renovascular disease, or those who may become pregnant.[6]

The national usage of ACE inhibitors has increased by 250% in the last five years. Captopril, the first ACE inhibitor prescribed for hypertension, is still significantly used, but the main growth in usage has been in enalapril and lisinopril. There is smaller, but increasing, usage in such drugs as ramipril, fosinopril and perindopril. Nationally the cost of ACE inhibitors has doubled to £192m per year in the last five years. The rising cost of ACE inhibitors is proportional to their rise in use, as the costs of the three main drugs used are broadly comparable. Currently there is a 2.4-fold variation in the use of these drugs by health authorities.[8]

Nitrates

The national usage of nitrates has increased by 25% in the past five years, although individual nitrate figures differ — the use of glyceryl trinitrate has remained relatively constant, there has been a small reduction in the use of isosorbide dinitrate and a substantial increase in the use of isosorbide mononitrate. The national annual cost of nitrates is now £60m and the trends in costs are broadly comparable with trends in usage. Glyceryl trinitrate is increasingly being prescribed as a spray and there has been a corresponding reduction in sublingual tablets and, more recently, in the patches and modified release tablets, which are expensive ways of prescribing glyceryl trinitrate. There has been a recent trend towards premium-priced modified release isosorbide mononitrate tablets. Currently there is a six-fold variation in health authority prescribing of these drugs.[8]

Calcium-channel blockers

Calcium-channel blockers have antihypertensive efficacy broadly similar to that of thiazides or β-blockers, although their safety during long-term treatment is less well established. They should therefore be considered for hypertension only when thiazides and β-blockers are contraindicated, not tolerated, or fail to control blood pressure.[6] The national usage of calcium-channel blockers has increased by 50% in the last five years with a trend towards higher doses and modified release preparations. Over this period of time nifedipine has remained constant and currently represents 50% usage. Amlodipine — which is marketed as a once-daily therapy — is now the next most widely used product, followed by diltiazem. The usage of verapamil has declined. The national cost of calcium-channel blockers has increased by 62% to £216m a year over the past five years. Currently there is a threefold variation in the use of these drugs by health authorities.[8]

Aspirin

Aspirin was first discovered to have anti-platelet properties 30 years ago; it acts to reduce thrombosis and prolong bleeding time. Clinical trials suggest that it should be used, unless contraindicated, to reduce cardiovascular morbidity and mortality in high-risk patients, such as those with coronary artery disease, post-MI and in some patients with atrial fibrillation. Low-dose aspirin is an inexpensive, effective and relatively safe therapy; the national prescribed usage has trebled in the past five years.

Lipid-lowering agents

Lipid-lowering agents are found within section 2.12 of the British National Formulary and fall into several groups. The main ones are statins and fibrates; the lesser groups include omega-3 fish oils, nicotinic acid derivatives, anion exchange resins and, recently, an ispaghula preparation.[6]

The Standing Medical Advisory Committee (SMAC) guidelines,[10] published last year with the Department of Health's executive letter, EL (97) 41,[11] have recently focused attention on the appropriate treatment selection for patients at risk from CHD. While numerous authors have questioned the details of the recommendations made in the SMAC report,[12] it is undoubtedly appropriate to target the use of therapeutic agents — such as the statins — where most benefit can be achieved. The SMAC guidelines refer to the Sheffield tables,[13] as a means of assessing CHD risks caused by different combinations of factors. It has been argued that the New Zealand risk tables are in practice easier to use and give a reasonable basis for assessing risks and deciding when to initiate therapy.[14] They also use the ratio of total cholesterol to high density lipoprotein (HDL), which may be a more effective means of measuring the risk of CHD than simple cholesterol levels. The SMAC guidelines also suggest an upper age limit of 70, primarily due to lack of evidence from trials of benefits to those aged over 70 for primary prevention of CHD.

The British National Formulary also provides a reminder that any lipid-lowering drug therapy must be combined with strict adherence to diet, maintenance of new ideal body weight and, if appropriate, reduction of blood pressure and cessation of smoking.[6] No major therapeutic decision, such as introducing a particular restrictive diet or lipid-lowering drugs, should be taken as a result of a single cholesterol determination. In those patients for whom drug therapy is being considered, at least two or three fasting measurements of cholesterol triglycerides and HDL cholesterol are necessary.

Prescriptions for lipid-lowering agents account for 4.7% of cardiovascular prescriptions and 17% of their cost; overall they account for over 3% of total prescribing costs.[8] It has also been estimated that the total cost of CHD is about 2.5% of the total National Health Service (NHS) budget.[15] The number of patient years represented by the prescriptions for statins is currently 500,000 using the World Health Organisation (WHO) Defined Daily Dose (DDD).[16] If the suggestions given in the SMAC guidelines — giving priority to secondary prevention — are followed, the additional costs to the NHS will clearly be substantial.

Statins

While prescribing for most of the groups of lipid-lowering drugs is static or declining, that of the statins is increasing rapidly, particularly since publication of the Scandinavian Simvastatin Survival Study (4S) study[5] at the end of 1994 and the West of Scotland Coronary Prevention Study (WOSCOPS) report in 1995.[3] The statins now account for over 75% of usage and 85% of costs of the lipid-lowering agents and the usage has increased nearly eightfold, from four million DDDs per quarter to over 31 million DDDs per quarter. Costs during the same period increased from £4m to £34m per quarter.[8]

Simvastatin currently accounts for 70% of all statin prescriptions, pravastatin for 14% and fluvastatin for 6%. Atorvastatin and cerivastatin are two new agents; atorvastatin already accounts for 7% of prescriptions and appears to be rapidly increasing.[8] There is, as yet, insufficient evidence available to assess the clinical significance of the increased effects of atorvastatin on lowering triglycerides, or its variable effects on HDL.

The WHO DDDs for statins other than simvastatin are probably higher than those typically used in England. For the two newer statins — atorvastatin and cerivastatin — the recommended BNF doses also appear to be higher than is shown in practice by an examination of actual prescriptions.[17] Is it better to treat more patients for a given total cost with a lower dose, such as is typically used at present, or fewer patients with a higher dose which has been proven in trials to be effective? Whilst the various trials have undoubtedly proved the efficacy of statins, the minimum effective dose is less clear.

There is considerable variation across health authorities in the usage of statins as measured by DDDs per 1,000 lipid-lowering specific therapeutic group age-sex related prescribing units (STARPUs).[18] The national average is about 340, but the range is between 200 and 725. Furthermore, there is no apparent correlation between CHD mortality rates (1994/5 data) and usage of statins;[19] some areas have high statin usage and low mortality rates and others have low statin usage and high mortality rates. Even if only the population over 65 is examined, the correlation between mortality figures for a health authority and the level of statin usage is minimal.[8]

Overall usage is highest in the North West and lowest in the West Midlands, despite the fact that CHD mortality rates are high in the West Midlands. They are medium to high in most of the North West, which tends to correlate with statin usage. However some parts of the South West and South East have low mortality rates but high statin usage. It might be argued that the high use of statins helped to prevent CHD. However, the latest mortality data available refers to 1994/5 and the mortality rates in the South West and South East were low at that time, before the large increase in statin usage in the wake of the 4S and WOSCOP trials.[2,3]

Geographical variations in the occurrence of CHD, in addition to the other risk factors discussed above should, therefore, also be considered when deciding on prescribing policies. Simvastatin is the most commonly used statin in all health authorities and, in most, pravastatin is the second most common; however atorvastatin already holds that position in a few.[8] In a sample of prescriptions recently dispensed, 53% were for men and 44% for women; the remaining 3% did not specify.[17] It is considered that women are just as likely to suffer from CHD as men, but usually later in life, typically when aged over 70, which is, in theory above the upper age recommended by SMAC. Currently there is a 3.6-fold variation in the use of these drugs by health authorities.[8]

Fibrates

Clofibrate, the first of this group, has been on the market for over 30 years. It is now, however, restricted for use to those patients who have had a cholecystectomy and, subsequently, declining. Other fibrates have been introduced more recently; bezafibrate remains the most commonly used one, but newer fibrates — such as fenofibrate and particularly ciprofibrate — have increased rapidly. Over the past five years there has been a 70% increase in fibrate usage, although it has now levelled off. Fibrates now account for 18% of prescriptions for lipid-lowering drugs, but only 10% of the costs.[8] There is evidence from trials that fibrates are effective; however, they have a lower popularity profile and appear very infrequently in the current major clinical trials.

Conclusion

CHD is caused by a variety of factors. There are a number of treatment methods currently available, but patients should also be encouraged to pursue healthy lifestyles, as part of general health promotion. Healthy eating, regular exercise, avoiding obesity and modest alcohol consumption are all beneficial. Older people have an intrinsically higher risk of CHD and, therefore, gain more benefit from health promotion programmes than younger adults.

References

1. The NHS Centre for Reviews and Dissemination. *Effective Healthcare bulletin*. York, 1998.

2. Randomized trial of cholesterol lowering in 4,444 patients with coronary heart disease: the Scandinavian Simvastatin Survival Study (4S). *Lancet* 1994; **344**: 1383–9.

3. Shepherd J, Cobbe SM, Ford I *et al*. Prevention of coronary heart disease with pravastatin in men with hyper-cholesterlaemia. *N Engl J Med* 1995; **333**: 1301–7.

4. The Health of the Nation briefing pack 1997. Department of Health.

5. Medical Research Council Working Party. MRC trial of treatment in mild hypertension. *BMJ* 1985; **291**: 97–104.

6. British National Formulary 1998 No 36. British Medical Association and Royal Pharmaceutical Society of Great Britain.

7. Wassertheil-Smoller S, Oberman A, Blaufox MD *et al*. The trial of antihypertensive interventions and management (TAIM) study. Final results with regard to blood pressure, cardiovascular risk, and quality of life. *Am J Hypertens* 1992; **5**: 37–44.

8. Prescribing analysis and cost (PACT) data 1998. Prescription pricing authority.

9. Sever P, Beevers G, Bulpitt C *et al*. Management guidelines in essential hypertension: report of the second working party of the British Hypertension Society. *BMJ* 1993; **306**: 983–7.

10. Standing medical advisory committee. *The use of statins*. London: 1997.

11. NHS Executive letter (EL (97)41). Statement on use of statins. Department of Health, 1997.

12. Correspondence, Use of statins; *BMJ* 1997; **315**: 1615–20.

13. Ramsey LE, Haq IU, Jackson PR, Yeo WW. The Sheffield table for primary prevention of coronary heart disease. *Lancet* 1996; **348**: 1251–2.

14. Published in a report on the management of mildly raised blood pressure. New Zealand Ministry of Health.

15. The Health of the Nation 1991. HMSO.

16. Guidelines for ATC clasification and DDD assignment 1996.

17. Sample of prescriptions, 1998. Prescription pricing authority.

18. Lloyd DC, Harris CM, Roberts DJ. Specific therapeutic group age-sex related prescribing units (STAR-PUs): weightings for analysing general practices' prescribing in England. *BMJ* 1995; **311**: 991–4.

19. Department of health public health common data set 1995. Institute of public health, University of Surrey.

Secondary prevention: economics

Caroline Morrison, Greater Glasgow Health Board, Glasgow

The first question to be addressed when determining the economics of secondary prevention of myocardial infarction (MI) is whether or not a therapy works. Thus, effectiveness is the primary issue to be considered before cost-effectiveness can be established.

Effectiveness of current therapies

Use of aspirin

Aspirin has been shown to be effective in preventing recurrent events in patients with previous MI and vascular events in those with stable and unstable angina.[1] There is a reduction over a two-year period of around 40 per 1,000 cases of MI, stroke or vascular death for post-MI patients, and a reduction of around 20 per 1,000 cases for those in other high-risk groups.[1]

Other antiplatelet therapies provide small, additional, benefit but are more expensive.

Use of β-blockers

β-blockers are effective in patients post MI, providing benefit of around 16-19 fewer deaths per 1,000 patients treated over a one-year period (*NNT*=48).[2,3] β-blockers have also been shown to reduce the number of cases of non-fatal MI from 7.5% to 5.6% over one year (*NNT*=56). The absolute benefit of β-blocker use is greater in older patients due to their higher initial risk of the condition. β-blockers are not contraindicated in those with heart failure – although careful use is required[4] – and are particularly beneficial in diabetic patients.[5] Their benefit in patients with stable angina has not been shown except in symptom management.

Hypertension control

Hypertension is a powerful risk factor for coronary events and stroke. Controlling hypertension is, therefore, important in secondary prevention – it continues to be a risk following MI if untreated.[6,7] Patients with existing coronary heart disease are treated with the same criteria as those without the disease. Studies carried out in general populations revealed that prolonged reduction of 7.5 mmHg diastolic pressure was associated with a 46% and 29% decrease in the risk of stroke and coronary heart disease, respectively.[8]

Maintenance of lipid levels

Management of lipids has become a popular topic of discussion since the publication of three secondary prevention statin trials: the Scandinavian Simvastatin Survival Study (4S),[9] the Cholesterol and Recurrent Events (CARE) trial[10] and the Long-term Intervention with Pravastatin in Ischaemic Disease (LIPID) study.[11] Although these studies comprise different groups of patients (ie post MI, angina, post-bypass surgery and coronary heart disease patients), each reveals a 25-30% reduction in coronary events in post MI and angina patients over a five-year period.

Smoking cessation

Modifying health-related behaviours, such as smoking, also has benefit in the secondary prevention of MI. Smoking cessation in observational studies indicates a reduction of 27 deaths per 1,000 patient years of cessation and a reduction to the level of non-smokers after three years.[12,13] Since smoking has been shown to be a powerful risk factor for incident coronary heart disease, it would seem counterintuitive to assume that smoking cessation following MI or unstable angina is beneficial, although the benefit may be different from that documented in observational studies.

Exercise

Exercise has a beneficial effect on the ability to exercise further and on physiological measures of cardiac disease; it also seems to have a beneficial effect on angina.[14] Although independent exercise has not indicated a significant effect on reinfarction, multifactorial rehabilitation programmes including exercise have been shown in meta-analyses to reduce mortality by 20-25% – no significant effect on non-fatal infarction, however, has been found.[15,16]

Individual rehabilitation programmes comprise different contents and modes of delivery, making it difficult to assess the effectiveness of each. Little evidence is currently available to determine which constituents and which manner of delivery are more effective than others – a recent randomized controlled trial, however, has indicated the benefits of three times per week aerobic training on cardiorespiratory fitness, psychological profiles, quality of life and vocational status.[17]

Another issue to be considered is the length of rehabilitation effectiveness. The perseverance with an exercise programme, smoking cessation or even dietary change is always problematical – how long support should be offered and whether or not the National Health Service (NHS) or others should fund long-term support are questions that need debate.

Diet

Modification of diet is also effective in secondary prevention.[18,19] This, however, should not be regarded solely in terms of lipid modification. Lipid-lowering drugs have been shown to have a complementary effect to lipid-lowering diets. The diet and reinfarction trial (DART) involved altering individuals' fat, fish and fibre intakes to determine whether or not diet had an effect on MI and death rates.[18] This trial showed a reduction of 29% in total mortality over two years by increasing oil-rich fish consumption although total cholesterol levels were not changed. Increasing fibre intake and possibly antioxidant intake, or other nutritional change, may provide benefit without changing lipid levels.

Cost-effectiveness of current therapies

There is a difference between the relative and absolute risk reduction of MI. A relative risk reduction of 30%, for instance, may mean an absolute risk reduction of 1% if the initial risk is 3%, but could mean an absolute risk reduction of 10% if the initial risk is 30%. The greater benefit is, obviously, in the latter.

Cost-effectiveness allows us to rank interventions in order of effectiveness per unit cost – thus, it involves the comparison of interventions. Such ranking and comparing of interventions is independent of available funding. If either the prevalence of a condition changes (altering the number of people eligible for an intervention) or the cost of an intervention changes, the cut-off point in the cost-effectiveness ranking, above which a service is provided and below which it is not, will need to change if overall costs are to stay the same.

The question, therefore, of which patients to target with effective therapies depends partly on the initial level of risk – those at highest risk gain greatest benefit – and also on the cost of therapies and the number of patients eligible.

One problem associated with secondary prevention of MI is that not all patients receive the necessary interventions. An example of this is seen in the use of statins. At almost all lipid levels, there is approximately a 30% benefit of treatment (although there may be a lower threshold of total blood lipid below which there is little or no benefit). However, cost-effectiveness increases as absolute risk – calculated by assessing other risk factors as well as lipid levels – increases. At what absolute risk level or cost-effectiveness level should patients be treated? Expenditure on statins has risen steeply since the publication of the three statin trials.[20] However, recent audits in Scotland have shown that cholesterol levels in 20-55% of coronary heart disease patients are poorly recorded, and that most remaining patients would be using a statin recommended by recent guidelines.[21–3] If equitable, complete, coverage of the population in terms of pharmacological lipid management was achieved, expenditure on statin use would double or treble. As the NHS funding sector for this area is stable, the question of which other treatments should not be funded to achieve this end must be considered.

One alternative is to raise the threshold for intervention. In addition, in lipid management there is evidence that many patients at low risk – even lower than current guidelines would recommend – are receiving statin therapy. Evidence shows that, in our own health authority, around 54% of statin prescribing is for the lowest dose. [Personal communicaton.] Given the range of cholesterol levels and the objectives set, it would not be possible for the targets to be reached with these low doses in most patients. This suggests that either doctors are not following advice on who should be treated or they are not reviewing patients who have been prescribed a statin to ensure the correct dose has been given and target levels achieved.

The Action on Secondary Prevention through Intervention to Reduce Events (ASPIRE) study, as well as other audits, has provided further evidence to confirm that secondary prevention interventions are applied in only a limited proportion of the coronary heart disease population.[24] ASPIRE was carried out in the UK and involved patients after elective percutaneous transluminal coronary angioplasty, coronary artery bypass surgery and acute MI, as well as those who had been admitted to hospital for acute myocardial ischaemia without infarction. These patients were recruited at least six months after the event. Approximately 20% of the participants were still smoking, 33% had a body mass index >30, 9% had a diastolic pressure >100 mmHg and 63% had total cholesterol >6 mmol/l. Aspirin use at follow-up ranged between <80% and >90% in different groups. Only about one-third of those post-infarct were using a β-blocker.

Similar results were shown in a primary care study carried out in Scotland, in which approximately 75% of patients were using aspirin and 14% had poorly-controlled blood pressure (>l60 mmHg systolic or 90 mmHg diastolic).[23]

Much money is currently being spent on therapies providing benefit in the future. Another economic problem regarding the cost-effective therapies is that these costs will fall mainly on primary care – principally nurses' time for monitoring risk factors and prescribing costs – while the benefits (in terms of money) will fall mainly on secondary care where reduced admissions should occur. It is difficult to transfer monies between these two healthcare sectors. The savings in secondary care, which flow from reduced admissions, are more apparent than real unless there is the potential to close a group of beds, eg a ward.

A recent study shows additional cost to be mostly in nurse time and statin-prescribing.[22] This study estimated that one bed day/year was saved for each patient in the intervention group. In a population of approximately 500,000, there is a potential for reducing bed-use by 13,700 bed days/year and subsequent closure of a number of beds if statistics prove to be correct in actual practice. There would still, however, remain the problem of transferring the savings from one healthcare sector to another. The other benefits of secondary prevention are intangibles: eg quality of life, increased life expectancy, improved symptoms and reduced burden on carers.

Conclusion

The economic problems in secondary prevention include determining how to:

- rank effective treatments and where to draw the cut-off point for cost-effectiveness funding
- persuade doctors to use the defined cut-off points and to establish improved methods of ensuring eligible patients receive interventions, as many more patients could benefit from optimum therapy
- fund the increased costs involved in using effective therapies more widely, in the knowledge that the benefits will be reaped in the future
- easily transfer resource from secondary to primary care.

Understanding these problems and accepting that there are difficulties, both in setting thresholds and obtaining agreement with clinicians about their use in clinical practice, is a step towards tackling the economic problems associated with secondary prevention.

References

1. Antiplatelet Trialists' Collaboration. Collaborative overview of randomised trials of antiplatelet therapy 1: Prevention of death, myocardial infarction, and stroke by prolonged antiplatelet therapy in various categories of patients. *BMJ* 1994; **308**: 81–106.

2. Yusuf S, Peto R, Lewis J *et al*. Beta-blockade during and after myocardial infarction: an overview of the randomized trials. *Prog Cardiovasc Dis* 1985; **27**: 335–71.

3. Held P, Yusuf S. Effects of beta-blockers and calcium channel blockers in acute myocardial infarction. *Eur Heart J* 1993; **14**: 18–25.

4. CIBIS II Investigators and Committees. The cardiac insufficiency bisoprolol study II: a randomised trial. *Lancet* 1999; **353**: 9–13.

5. Kendall MJ, Lynch KP, Hjalmarson A, Kjekshus J. *Ann Intern Med* 1995; **123**: 358–67.

6. Wong ND, Cupples LA, Ostfeld AM *et al*. Risk factors for long-term coronary prognosis after initial myocardial infarction: The Framingham Study. *Am J Epidemiol* 1989; **130**: 469–80.

7. Connolly DC, Elveback LR, Oxman HA. Coronary heart disease in Rochester, Minnesota 1950–1975. Effect of hypertension and its treatment on survival of patients with coronary artery disease. *Mayo Clin Proc* 1983; **58**: 248–54.

8. MacMahon S, Peto R, Cutler J *et al*. Blood pressure, stroke and coronary heart disease. Part 1, prolonged differences in blood pressure: prospective observational studies corrected for the regression dilution bias. *Lancet* 1990; **335**: 765–74.

9. Scandinavian Simvastatin Survival Study Group. Randomized trial of cholesterol lowering in 444 patients with coronary heart disease; the Scandinavian Simvastatin Survival Study (4S). *Lancet* 1994; **344**: 1383–9.

10. Sacks FM, Pfeffer MA, Moye LA *et al*, for the Cholesterol and Recurrent Events trial Investigators. The effect of pravastatin on coronary events after myocardial infarction in patients with average cholesterol levels. *N Engl J Med* 1996; **335**: 1001–9.

11. The Long-Term Intervention with Pravastatin in Ischaemic Disease (LIPID) Study Group. Prevention of cardiovascular events and death with pravastatin in patients with coronary heart disease and a broad range of initial cholesterol levels. *N Engl J Med* 1998; **339**: 1349–57.

12. Wilhelmsson L. Coronary heart disease epidemiology of smoking and intervention studies of smoking. *Am Heart J* 1988; **115**: 242–9.

13. Daly LE, Mulcahy R, Graham IM, Hickey N. Long-term effect of mortality of stopping smoking after unstable angina and myocardial infarction. *BMJ* 1983; **287**: 324–6.

14. Wenger NK, Froelicher ES, Smith LK *et al*. *Cardiac rehabilitation as secondary prevention*. Rockville, Maryland: Agency for Health Care Policy and Research and National Heart, Lung and Blood Institute, 1995.

15. Oldridge NB, Guyatt GH, Fischer ME *et al*. Cardiac rehabilitation after myocardial infarction. Combined experience of randomized clinical trials. *JAMA* 1988; **260**: 945–50.

16. O'Connor GT, Buring JE, Yusuf S *et al*. An overview of randomized trials of rehabilitation with exercise after myocardial infarction. *Circulation* 1989; **80**: 234–44.

17. Dugmore LD, Tipson RJ, Philips MH *et al*. Changes in cardiorespiratory fitness, psychological wellbeing, quality of life and vocational status following a 12-month cardiac exercise rehabilitation programme. *Heart* 1999; **81**: 359–66.

18. Burr ML, Fehily AM, Gilbert JF *et al*. Effects of changes in fat, fish and fibre intakes on death and myocardial reinfarction: diet and reinfarction trial (DART). *Lancet* 1989; **2**: 757–61.

19. De Lorgeril M, Renaud S, Mamelle N *et al*. Mediterranean alpha-linoleic acid-rich diet in secondary prevention of coronary heart disease. *Lancet* 1994; **343**: 1454–9.

20. Pharmacy Practice Division of the Common Services Agency. *National Health Service in Scotland Quarterly Bulletin*. Scottish Office of the Department of Health, 1998.

21. McKinlay JJ, Short AD. An audit of secondary prevention in patients with established coronary heart disease. *Health Bull* 1998; **56**: 592–602.

22. Campbell NC, Thain J, Deans HG *et al*. Secondary prevention clinics for coronary heart disease: randomized trial of effect on health. *BMJ* 1998; **316**:1434–7.

23. Campbell NC, Thain J, Deans HG *et al*. Secondary prevention in coronary heart disease: baseline survey of provision in general practice. *BMJ* 1998; **316**: 1430–4.

24. ASPIRE Steering Group. A British Cardiac Society survey on the potential for secondary prevention of coronary disease: ASPIRE (Action on secondary prevention through intervention to reduce events) - principal results. *Heart* 1996; **75**: 334–42.

Index